SpringerBriefs in Psychology

SpringerBriefs present concise summaries of cutting-edge research and practical applications across a wide spectrum of fields. Featuring compact volumes of 50 to 125 pages, the series covers a range of content from professional to academic. Typical topics might include:

- A timely report of state-of-the-art analytical techniques
- A bridge between new research results as published in journal articles and a contextual literature review
- A snapshot of a hot or emerging topic
- An in-depth case study or clinical example
- A presentation of core concepts that readers must understand to make independent contributions

SpringerBriefs in Psychology showcase emerging theory, empirical research, and practical application in a wide variety of topics in psychology and related fields. Briefs are characterized by fast, global electronic dissemination, standard publishing contracts, standardized manuscript preparation and formatting guidelines, and expedited production schedules.

More information about this series at http://www.springer.com/series/10143

Sabine Bährer-Kohler • Blanca Bolea-Alamanac
Editors

Diversity in Global Mental Health

Gender, Lifespan, Access to Care,
Treatment and Social Strata

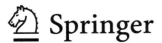 Springer

Editors
Sabine Bährer-Kohler
Dr. Bährer-Kohler & Partners
Basel, Switzerland

International University of Catalonia
Tropical Neurology and Neuroinfection
Master
Barcelona, Spain

Blanca Bolea-Alamanac
Centre for Addiction and Mental Health
University of Toronto
Toronto, ON, Canada

ISSN 2192-8363   ISSN 2192-8371   (electronic)
SpringerBriefs in Psychology
ISBN 978-3-030-29111-2   ISBN 978-3-030-29112-9   (eBook)
https://doi.org/10.1007/978-3-030-29112-9

This Springer imprint is published by the registered company Springer Nature Switzerland AG
The registered company address is: Gewerbestrasse 11, 6330 Cham, Switzerland

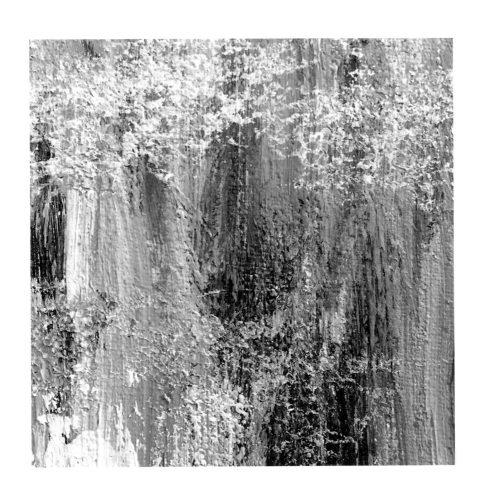

Foreword

John Snow was one of the fathers of public health, one of the first epidemiologists, and the one who debunked the miasma theory. Investigating the 1854 London Cholera Outbreak, he established some fundamental principles of public health: he looked for an underlying theme that linked the infected patients together. He examined the neighborhood. He gathered all relevant information about the outbreak. He talked to everyone he could. He produced a geographical map of cholera cases. He finally identified a water pump to be responsible for the outbreak. He then presented his findings to the local council who acted in removing the pump handle.

While our public health techniques have advanced, the principles remain. We are looking for underlying causes, we try to understand people's behaviors, we collect as much relevant information about the conditions in which the diseases we investigate spread, and we look for efficacious ways of how to stop or prevent their further spread and, fundamentally, how to promote the health of the public.

Removing a handle from a water pump, one can argue, is a simple action to stop the spread of a disease. Addressing mental health is certainly more complex as the causes are often manifold, and the best strategies of how to improve and achieve equity in mental health for all people worldwide require more than just one resolute action by a local council. It fundamentally requires action that influences the conditions in which people are born, grow, work, and age. Effective public health work to address mental health requires the identification of the specific health-determining societal factors in a given population. As these factors are often determined by policies, it requires to identify policy options that address these societal factors or, as some like to call them, the root causes.

In the case of the London Cholera Outbreak, they found a contaminated diaper in the water pipe. The root cause of course was not a diaper but an inappropriate open sewage system. This and other contamination cases finally lead to actions on increased sanitation.

This publication therefore unfolds the underlying themes of global mental health: diversity, gender, and life stages. Effective strategies to advance global mental health imply creating a culture of knowledge about sociocultural paradigms, working locally, accepting and promoting grassroots movements, and recognizing and appreciating differences and similarities across genders, cultures, societies, languages, and ethnicities.

Gender inequalities, discrimination, neglect, and stigma all pose challenges and barriers in caring for people with mental health problems and thus compromise their right to health.

The role that public health needs to play is to advocate, mediate, and enable: speaking up where inequities exist, where people are left behind, helping to find compromise between diverse cultural backgrounds, and enabling communities to appreciate differences so that they enrich – and not endanger – people's lives.

Addressing the root causes of ill-health, be it in the areas of mental health or communicable disease, requires skills to reach out beyond the medical services provided by the health care system. And it requires knowledge about those underlying factors that have a critical influence on people's health. This publication sheds some bright light on the latter.

Dr. Rüdiger Krech
Director, Health Promotion
Division of Universal Health Coverage and Healthier Populations
World Health Organization
Geneva, Switzerland

Foreword

Mental health conditions are pervasive. They can occur at all places and at all times throughout the world. There are no known universal foolproof protections for anybody against mental health conditions – age, gender, social status, race/ethnicity, and other factors. In other words, mental illness is no respecter of persons but just anybody can suffer from any form of mental illness at any time anywhere.

The direct and indirect costs of mental health conditions are hardly quantifiable.

It is common knowledge that especially in developing countries, there is a historical focus on communicable and more immediately life-threatening diseases such as infections including HIV/AIDS, viral hemorrhagic fevers, typhoid, malaria, etc. Partly for this reason, mental health conditions have often been overlooked as a public health issue, yet mental ill-health has profound effects on an individual's quality of life, physical and social well-being, and economic productivity.

Mental health conditions have great adverse personal, family, regional, and global effects.

Unfortunately, it can safely be said that mental health conditions have not by any stretch of the imagination received the desired attention anywhere in the world.

Throughout history most efforts to improve global mental health have focused on improving care for individuals living with psychological disorders, but the World Health Organization (WHO) stresses that a comprehensive definition of mental health should extend beyond the absence or presence of diagnosable psychological disorders to include "subjective well-being, perceived self-efficacy, autonomy, competence, intergenerational dependence and recognition of the ability to realize one's intellectual and emotional potential" [1].

Government and non-governmental organizations have attempted to put up efforts to address the issue of mental health conditions. The World Health Organization plays a key role and a few years ago developed the Mental Health Action Gap Action Programme (mhGAP) to address the need in closing the gap between mental health needs and access, largely through some kind of task shifting and task sharing.

In general common mental disorders are known to be highly prevalent globally, affecting people across all regions of the world. The argument of WHO is that mental, neurological, and substance use disorders are common in all regions of the world, affecting every community and age group across all income countries. It is further argued that while 14% of the global burden of disease is attributed to mental health disorders, most of the people affected (over 75%) in many low-income countries do not have access to the treatment they need.

The World Federation for Mental Health (WFMH) had existed before the mhGAP.

In fact the WFMH, an international membership organization, was founded in 1948 to advance, among all peoples and nations, the prevention of mental and emotional disorders, the proper treatment and care of those with such disorders, and the promotion of mental health. The organization has had a mission to promote the advancement of mental health awareness, prevention of mental disorders, advocacy, and best practice recovery-focused interventions all over the world. The specific goals of WFMH include heightening public awareness about the importance of mental health with the gaining of understanding and improving attitudes about mental disorders. In addition WFMH aims to promote mental health and prevent mental disorders and improve the care, treatment, and recovery of people with mental disorders [2].

In an ideal situation, global and cultural mental health should work to improve mental health and reduce mental ill-health especially in low-resource settings and among much more other vulnerable populations nationally and internationally. Strengthening leadership and building capacity in both government and non-government sectors to develop mental health and social support services that are high quality, equitable, and affordable and that protect the human rights of people with mental ill-health is a noble goal worthy of world attention.

Access to quality mental health care and awareness cannot be divorced from research and systems development, learning and teaching, and engagement with key stakeholders in the field of mental health in every community.

I will argue that worldwide, persons with mental disorders constitute a vulnerable group, whichever way the concept of vulnerability is construed.

The diversity of mental disorders in different genders and the apparent neglect of gender, age, and other psychosocial factors over another are reflected in the feminist theory [3]. Mental health knowledge and access differ in males and females and different age groups in many parts of the world. The ideas of gender roles, race, sexuality, and class strongly inform and perpetuate how people understand mental health. Access to mental health services differs in males and females in many parts of the world. This calls for mental health activism, which should be largely centered on the idea that people should all be able to make informed decisions about what to do with their mental health.

Recent developments in information and communications technology have given rise to the famous assertion that the world is now a global village. There are different operational understandings of globalization. Strictly speaking globalization is the free movement of goods, services, and people across the world in a seamless and integrated manner.

It has been argued that "globalization is grounded in the theory of comparative advantage, which implies that countries that are good at producing a particular good are better off exporting it to countries that are less efficient at producing that good. The corollary is that the latter country can then export the goods that it produces in an efficient manner to the former country which might be deficient in the same. The underlying assumption here is that not all countries are good at producing all sorts of goods/services and hence they benefit by trading with one another.

Globalization describes the growing interdependence of the world's economies, cultures, and populations, brought about by cross-border trade in goods and services, technology, and flows of investment, people, and information. Countries have built economic partnerships to facilitate these movements over many centuries" [4].

Globalization is linked to global health, including mental health.

Global health is the health of populations in a global context, transcending perspectives and concerns of individual nations. The whole philosophy lies on tackling the most important health problems globally based on equity and ethics of health as human rights.

Global mental health comes to the fore. The global mental health initiative works to establish a network of individuals and organizations with the aim of improving services for people living with mental ill-health and psychosocial disabilities worldwide, especially in low- and middle-income countries where effective services are oftentimes scarce and inefficient.

The global mental health initiative calls for health organizations and researchers to prioritize global mental health. Prof. Vikram Patel once said: "Global Health emphasizes global learning; thus while international health was built on the tradition of what the 'developed world' could teach those in the developing world, global health emphasizes what all countries can learn from one another and do together to address the health of all people who must share our planet" [5].

There is thus a clear overlap between the works of WHO, WFMH, and the recent Global Mental Health Movement. Yet there is a yawning need for synergy between these organizations and governments.

Have these developments translated to better and quality mental health awareness, access, and service worldwide? I do not think that current research findings will answer in the affirmative. If that is the case, what barriers may be attributable to the non-achievement of such laudable ventures and goals?

There is no doubt that dissemination is one crucial factor.

The new brief *Diversity and Global Mental Health: Gender, Lifespan, Access to Care, Treatment and Social Strata* edited by Prof. Baehrer-Kohler and Prof. Bolea-Alamanac has eloquently attempted to fill this gap.

The editors have carefully selected eminent scholars and experts in the field to do justice to the goal of this laudable venture.

A readable, handy text the eight chapters have captured and encapsulated all that is necessary for global distribution.

After the introduction the second chapter discusses the differences in prevalence of mental health with the inclusion of diversity, gender, and lifespan. The third chapter discusses the aspects of diversity and lifespan, while the fourth chapter delves into the issue of women, gender diversities, and mental health.

Diversity and gender differences in treatment together with global mental health services and access to care are key features which this brief has perfectly addressed. Oftentimes politics is at the epicenter of all successful programs, and this work has given sufficient attention to this all-important issue.

The value and merit of a material are not measured by the physical size but the content. This small brief is like a mental health scientific encyclopedia, soundly and scientifically taking on the fields of global health/mental health/neuroscience/gender/pharmacological and psychological treatments/biomedicine. The major thrust of this gold mine is to promote global mental health engagement and to improve quality of mental health care.

This *Diversity in Global Mental Health* prepared in such a manner that it is easy to read and quite affordable to the masses offers condensed scientific data, aimed at an audience that has limited time to process more detailed and expansive, often unnecessary, information. In this day and age when most people are pressed with time, with much to read, the approach of this new booklet is its own letter of recommendation to everyone.

The brief is a must-read for all health and mental health professionals and trainees, students, and faculty and serves as a ready reference tool for advanced researchers and practitioners alike.

While commending and congratulating the authors and editors on this innovative approach to writing, I am delighted to recommend this brief to everyone who shares the vision of good health and mental health – professionals and nonprofessionals alike.

Richard Uwakwe
Faculty of Medicine, Nnamdi Azikiwe University
Awka, Anambra State, Nigeria
December 26, 2018

References

1. WHO- World Health Organization. (2003). *Investing in mental health.* http://apps.who.int/iris/bitstream/handle/10665/87232/9789241564618_eng.pdf;jsessionid=20C18B6E31F9E9947DB7606780766EDF?sequence=1. 10th of Dec 2018
2. Health WffM. (2018). https://wfmh.global/. Accessed 10th of Dec 2018.
3. Mowbray, C. T., Herman, S. E., & Hazel, K. L. (1992). GENDER AND SERIOUS MENTAL ILLNESS: A Feminist Perspective. *Psychology of Women Quarterly, 16*(1):107–126. https://doi.org/10.1111/j.1471-6402.1992.tb00243.x
4. Economics PIfI. (2018). *What is globalization? And how has the global economy shaped the United States?* https://piie.com/microsites/globalization/what-is-globalization.html. Accessed tenth of Dec 2018.
5. Patel, V. (2014). Why mental health matters to global health. *Transcultural Psychiatry, 51*(6):777–789. https://doi.org/10.1177/1363461514524473.

Acknowledgments

We would like to extend our deepest gratitude to the publishers and all co-authors for their outstanding contributions and for their kind cooperation in bringing together this book.

Special thanks should be given to our families for their patience, understanding, and invaluable support.

Contents

Chapter 1
Introduction

Blanca Bolea-Alamanac and Sabine Bährer-Kohler

1.1 Why Is this Book Needed?

Humanity is both unique and diverse. Humans have populated the world and created a kaleidoscopic mosaic of societies, cultures, ethnicities, languages and beliefs. Different cultures have achieved different solutions to similar problems while at the same time all of us appear to agree to some basic truths. These are enshrined in the Universal Declaration of Human Rights [1] and in the international institutions that promote global human welfare by applying these principles. The World Health Organization is a specialized agency established on the seventh of April 1948 with the aim of directing and coordinating international health initiatives within the United Nations [2]. Initially most of these international programs focused on communicable diseases, as the organization developed, the importance of mental health was recognized as a priority. The definition of health which is universally learned by students in the health sciences worldwide acknowledges this fact: "Health is a state of complete physical, mental and social well-being and not merely the absence of disease or infirmity" [2]. Promoting mental health is the key in order to produce healthier societies. Several programs described in this book (such as mhgap—Chap. 7) were born out of international collaborations supported by the World Health Organization. Global mental health can be defined as "the area of study, research and practice that places a priority on improving mental health and achieving equity in mental health for all people worldwide" [3]. The objectives of this initiative cannot be achieved without ensuring implementation of human rights, eradication of poverty and social

B. Bolea-Alamanac (✉)
University of Toronto/Centre for Addiction and Mental Health, Toronto, ON, Canada

S. Bährer-Kohler
Dr. Bährer-Kohler & Partner, Basel, Switzerland

International University of Catalonia (UIC), Barcelona, Spain

© The Author(s) 2019
S. Bährer-Kohler, B. Bolea-Alamanac (eds.), *Diversity in Global Mental Health*,
SpringerBriefs in Psychology, https://doi.org/10.1007/978-3-030-29112-9_1

inequality and equality across ethnicities and genders. Effectively promoting mental health implies creating a culture of knowledge about sociocultural paradigms, working locally, accepting and promoting grassroots movements and recognizing differences and similarities across genders, cultures, societies, languages and ethnicities. Some authors [4, 5] have criticized the discipline of global mental health as a type of medical colonization. This criticism must be acknowledged and acted upon. There is evidence that effective and sustainable mental health interventions require cultural adaptation and local support [6]. The voices of those who ultimately use, deliver or support the service in the field must be heard. Interventions that grow organically from the society where they are rooted should be supported. This does not necessarily mean that international collaborations should not be encouraged. Different societies may find points in common and can benefit from synergic effects arising from the experience of shared challenges. This expertise can be translated and adapted to new environments. Furthermore, international cooperation is essential to find proactive solutions for specific populations such as war refugees, to act in emergency situations or when a lengthy consultation process is not feasible, to research the biology of mental illness and to develop effective pharmacological treatments. This book is a concise compendium of the basic concepts and actions required to effectively promote global mental health. It is necessary because as communication improves and networks become global, new challenges arise that require world-wide solutions. Finding common goals to work towards is crucial and this book summarizes the background and action points required to implement effective programs and promote mental health globally. The editors have partnered with academics and researchers working in the field worldwide in order to obtain a diverse view. A 'booklet' format was agreed as it was considered the most efficient conduct for the audience we wanted to reach. In a world where time is precious, we set ourselves the task of summarizing scientific research with a pragmatic focus, highlighting those key aspects that can infer change and favouring synthesis over breadth.

1.2   Definition of Diversity

Diversity is generally defined as the property of being composed by different elements [7]. When referring to the human condition it is defined as the inclusion of different types of people (such as different races or cultures) in a group or organizational structure [7]. Humans are diverse by nature. Exposure to a variety of environments has forced the human brain to adapt by developing different languages, customs, philosophies, political systems and beliefs. The ability to adapt is one of humanity's strengths and is the consequence of having a complex central nervous system that requires years to reach maturity. This same system can fall ill in unique and sophisticated ways specific to humans and difficult to replicate in animal models. What makes us human is paradoxically also one of the greatest threats to our own health. Mental illness is universal, but how it manifests is heavily coloured by ethnicity, environment, culture and gender. This has been beautifully depicted over the ages by artists and academics, from the first descriptions of depression and anxiety in Babylonian texts circa 1894–1595 BC [8], to contemporaneous academic publications detailing the circumstances and consequences of mental illness and their corresponding artistic expressions in art and literature. Mental illness has been identified and explained differently by various cultures ranging from being the product of incantations and witchcraft to a gift from the gods. Before the twentieth century, and in the absence of effective treatments, these beliefs where the only guide for many individuals suffering from mental health problems and their families. Cultural and spiritual doctrines played a key role in how these individuals were treated, sometimes offering compassion and care, oftentimes ostracizing and expulsing them to the periphery of society [9]. The interaction of cultural diversity and illness cannot be ignored. New services and programs should take into account this diversity from the early design stages to the final execution process providing flexibility and cultural adaptations where required.

1.3 Definition of Gender

Gender differs from sex in that it is not just a biological construct, but a concept based on cultural and societal norms. When referring strictly to the biological aspects the word 'sex' is generally preferred. Gender differences abound in society. Despite efforts to achieve equality across genders, this is arguably one of the greatest equality gaps in modern society. The movement underpinning gender equality, commonly known as 'feminism' has also undergone several revisions with perhaps the majority of scholars supporting an intersectional view. Intersectional feminism is based on the concept that gender discrimination is intertwined with other patterns of social injustice and ingrained in cultural, racial and ethnic inequity [10]. From this perspective, gender equality cannot be achieved if other types of discrimination are not addressed simultaneously. This movement acknowledges that individuals can be subjected to several types of oppression at the same time. It is this network of social inequities that ultimately affects individuals and society at large negatively, producing, for example, poorer health outcomes for individuals or communities affected by these patterns of discrimination.

1.4 Lifespan Factors

A universal factor affecting health is age. Our world is getting older, improvements in public health and medical technology have allowed us to live longer and healthier. However, this entails new challenges. More complex healthcare systems are required to assist the elderly. Long term housing solutions and stable financial support is also needed. Age-related discrimination is an emerging issue. Healthy elderly individuals are excluded from job opportunities and often discriminated financially. For those who cannot live independently, their care falls mostly on women, often relatives, who are not paid but required to do this work. This adds another dimension of complexity to aging as it affects other strata of society at their point of maximum productivity. Complex health systems solutions are required to deal with an aging society. These include promotion of home care, prevention of common causes of comorbidity in the elderly (such as prevention of falls and infections), monitoring of premorbid states (such as incipient cognitive deterioration) and the promotion of healthy aging [11].

1.5   Reducing Stigma

Stigma is traditionally defined as a mark of disgrace or disapproval with a person, a particular context or a set of circumstances [12]. When applied to mental health, it refers to a group of factors colluding together within a power relational system leading to discrimination of individuals with mental illness [13]. These factors include but are not limited to: loss of status, stereotyping, social isolation, labelling and other forms of discrimination [13]. Stigma is not restricted to the individual and interpersonal level, it can be structural as well. Structural stigma is based on two main pillars: discriminatory institutional policies (including laws) and social dominance of specific cultural norms in the detriment of others [14]. Stigma is one of the main factors precluding individuals with mental health difficulties accessing care. Social stigma has been used to decrease funding opportunities for mental health services [15], as patients are not as likely to lobby against changes as other populations. Until recently, some cultures considered mental health problems as a family issue which could not be discussed outside the home. This led to an 'invisible' burden of disease generating severe intergenerational effects that perpetuated poor health. Interventions to reduce stigma are necessary. Effective eradication of stigma requires a multifaceted approach. Education both about mental illness and treatment is important as well as promotion of a healthy understanding of mental health from childhood to adulthood. Changes in laws, directives or policies that discriminate against people with mental illness is also necessary. Special safeguards and protections may be required such as strict confidentiality procedures and open-door policies for patients accessing services. Battling stigma may require partnering with medical and non-medical organizations, wide networking and the creation of new structures of support for people affected by mental illness. Special attention should be given to the portrayal of mental health and mental illness in the media. Negative stereotypes can be perpetuated this way when the same channels can be used to disseminate accurate information and promote mental wellbeing.

1.6 Outline of this Booklet

This booklet is meant to be used both as a summary of knowledge and a guide for further resources in the emerging field of global mental health with a particular focus on the challenges of diversity, gender and lifespan. The second chapter is a concise introduction to the epidemiology of psychiatric illness. Chapter 3 reviews how gender, life stages and diversity affect mental health delineating challenges and opportunities for the promotion of wellness. Chapter 4 focuses on the interplay between gender and cultural diversity. Chapter 5 summarizes current and past research challenges as regards to the development of treatments through the lenses of gender and diversity and proposes new ways of including previously marginalized populations in research. Chapter 6 reviews barriers to access care and outlines the changes and strategies required to address those. Chapter 7 is a case study of a successful collaboration to provide mental health care to a vulnerable population (emigrants in the Mexico-US border) situated in the broader context of Global Mental Health promotion. Finally, Chapter 8 elaborates on the junction of governance, diplomacy, policy and mental health, providing a guide for further reading as well as an outline of the main action points required at a political level to improve mental health globally.

In summary, this booklet is an extensive introduction to a wide and developing topic: Global Mental Health. It is written by a range of experts, working worldwide to improve mental health at a global level. The editors are sure that this booklet will contribute to the development of the field as well as encourage local, national and international efforts to battle mental illness and stigma, and to promote global mental health around the world.

References

1. United Nations-General Assembly. (1949). *Universal declaration of human rights*. Department of State publication; 3381., vol Accessed from https://nla.gov.au/nla.cat-vn33809. U.S. Govt. Print. Off, Washington.
2. World Health Organization. (1948). *Constitution of the World Health Organization: Principles*. https://www.who.int/about/mission/en/. Accessed 24 January 2019.
3. Patel, V., & Prince, M. (2010). Global mental health: A new global health field comes of age. *JAMA, 303*(19), 1976–1977.
4. Mills, C. (2014). Globalising mental health or pathologising the global south? Mapping the ethics. *Theory and Practice of Global Mental Health, 1*.
5. Wessells, M. (2015). *Decolonizing global mental health: The psychiatrization of the majority world by China Mills*. New York: Routledge, 2014. 175 pp. $48.95 (paper). ISBN 978-1-84872-160-9, vol 59.
6. Healey, P., Stager, M. L., Woodmass, K., Dettlaff, A. J., Vergara, A., Janke, R., & Wells, S. J. (2017). Cultural adaptations to augment health and mental health services: A systematic review. *BMC Health Services Research, 17*(1), 8.
7. Merriam-Webster Incorporated. (2004). *The Merriam-Webster Dictionary*. Merriam-Webster, Incorporated.

  8. Reynolds, E. H., & Kinnier Wilson, J. V. (2014). Neurology and psychiatry in Babylon. *Brain, 137*(9), 2611–2619.
  9. Dilling, H., Thomsen, H. P., & Hohagen, F. (2010). Care of the insane in Lubeck during the 17th and 18th centuries. *History of Psychiatry, 21*(84 Pt 4), 371–386.
 10. Rogers, J., & Kelly, U. A. (2011). Feminist intersectionality: Bringing social justice to health disparities research. *Nursing Ethics, 18*(3), 397–407.
 11. World Health Organization. (2015). https://www.who.int/ageing/healthy-ageing/en/. Accessed 18 Feb 2019.
 12. Stevenson, A. (2010). *Oxford Dictionary of English*.
 13. Buchter, R. B., & Messer, M. (2017). Interventions for reducing self-stigma in people with mental illnesses: A systematic review of randomized controlled trials. *German Medical Science: GMS e-journal, 15*.
 14. Hatzenbuehler, M. L. (2016). Structural stigma: Research evidence and implications for psychological science. *The American Psychologist, 71*(8), 742–751.
 15. Corrigan, P. W., Markowitz, F. E., & Watson, A. C. (2004). Structural levels of mental illness stigma and discrimination. *Schizophrenia Bulletin, 30*(3), 481–491.

Chapter 2
Differences in Prevalence of Mental Health with the Inclusion of Diversity, Gender and Lifespan

Francisco Javier Carod Artal

Key Points

- Mental health disorders are frequent. Estimated prevalence of common mental health disorders range between 3.8% (substance abuse), 5.4% (mood disorders) and 6.7% (anxiety disorders).
- Data from meta-analysis of epidemiological studies showed that nearly one in five survey respondents (17.6%) met criteria for a common mental health disorder during the previous 12 months and 29% met lifetime prevalence for mental health disorders.
- Mental health disorders are one of the main causes of disease burden worldwide and account for a significant percentage of years lived with disability.
- Vulnerable groups at increased risk of mental health problems include women, ethnic and sexual minorities, refugees, asylum-seekers, offenders, individuals with addiction problems, the homeless, and people with physical and/or learning disabilities.
- Gender is a determinant of mental health, and gender differences significantly affect the prevalence rate of common mental disorders. Gender differences also occur in age of symptom onset, course of the disease, frequency of symptoms, and long-term outcomes.

(continued)

F. J. C. Artal (✉)
Neurology Department, Raigmore Hospital, Inverness, UK

Research Unit, Health Science Center, Inverness, UK

Universitat International of Catalunya (UIC), Barcelona, Spain
e-mail: javier.carodartal@nhs.net

© The Author(s) 2019
S. Bährer-Kohler, B. Bolea-Alamanac (eds.), *Diversity in Global Mental Health*,
SpringerBriefs in Psychology, https://doi.org/10.1007/978-3-030-29112-9_2

- Gender-related risk factors that significantly affect women include socio-economic inequality, lower social status, and gender-based violence among others.
- Epidemiological studies reported a sex ratio (women: men) of 2.1 for lifetime and 1.7 for point prevalence of major depressive disorder in adults. Women have a higher lifetime prevalence of mood and anxiety disorders than men, and a later onset of psychoses. There is a female preponderance within the internalising spectrum which includes depression, anxiety, and eating, post-traumatic stress and somatoform disorders.
- Men have greater rates of substance dependence, alcohol abuse and anti-social personality disorder.
- Mental disorders are also common in the elderly, and 15% of the population above 60 suffers depression or dementia, and 4% anxiety disorders.
- Although meta-analyses of population studies have provided aggregated estimates for the prevalence of most common mental disorders, a substantial inter-survey heterogeneity and data variability exists.

2.1 Introduction

Mental health and substance use disorders are common, widespread, can be disabling and often remain untreated. Common mental health disorders are mood (depression and bipolar disorder), and anxiety disorders including panic disorder, obsessive/compulsive disorder, and post-traumatic stress disorder (PTSD) [1].

Research in epidemiology of mental health and mental illness was favoured by the development and implementation of specific diagnostic criteria since the late 1970s [2]. Following the publication of the *Diagnostic and Statistical Manual of Mental Disorders*, Third Edition, (DSM-III) a large body of epidemiological research accumulated in the last three decades [1]. A rapid growth in the number of mental health epidemiological studies provided population estimates (period and lifetime prevalence) of some common mental health disorders.

However, several gaps in our knowledge remain and the relative proportion of prevalence studies about mental health disorders in developing countries and ethnic minorities is low. In addition, a gender bias in research has been noted (see Chap. 4), and the proportion of studies about the differential impact of mental disorders in women, ethnic and other minorities is noticeably smaller. In this chapter, differences in prevalence of mental health with the inclusion of diversity, gender and lifespan will be reviewed.

2.2 Review

2.2.1 Mental Health Prevalence

The Global burden of Disease 1990–2010 Study estimated that worldwide around 400 million people suffered from depression, 272 million from anxiety and 140 million people had alcohol or drug abuse disorder [3]. Approximately 80 million children worldwide have some type of behavioural disorder [3].

Global prevalence of common mental health disorders has been evaluated in a systematic review and meta-analysis of 174 surveys across 63 countries that provided period and lifetime prevalence estimates. Pooled period prevalence of mood disorders across 148 surveys was 5.4% with a lifetime prevalence of 9.6%. For anxiety disorders, pooled period and lifetime prevalence were respectively 6.7% and 12.9%. Substance use disorders had a pooled period prevalence of 3.8% [2]. In addition, nearly one in five survey respondents (17.6%) met criteria for a common mental health disorder during the previous 12 months and 29% met lifetime prevalence for any mental health disorder [2].

Data from the Global Burden of Disease Study found that mental and substance use disorders were the fifth leading disorder category of global disability-adjusted life years (DALYS) and accounted for 183.9 million DALYs in 2010 [4]. In addition, mental and substance use disorders were the leading cause of years lived with disability (YLD) worldwide (23%) [4].

The 2013 Global Burden of Disease study reported that depression alone was the second leading cause of YLD, followed by lower back pain [5]. Depression was the most common mental health disorder followed by anxiety, schizophrenia and bipolar disorder. Severe mental health disorders are linked with higher rates of disability and mortality, and people with major depression or schizophrenia have a 40–60% greater chance of premature death when compared to healthy individuals [1, 6].

It has been estimated that by 2030, mental health problems and depression in particular will be the leading cause of mortality and morbidity globally, whereas in 1990 depression was the fourth largest contributor to disease burden [1]. Furthermore, the burden of mental and substance abuse disorders increased by 37% during the period 1990–2010, and this rise was driven by population growth and aging [4].

2.2.2 Diversity

Culture plays a significant role in the understanding of mental health, and different cultures perceive mental health in a different way. Treatment-seeking patterns may also vary across cultures and people from ethnic minorities are less likely to seek mental health support or treatment. Other factors such as racism, discrimination and cultural stereotyping may also bias epidemiological studies [7]. The DSM-5 cultural formulation interview recommended considering cultural factors influencing patient's perspectives about symptoms and therapeutic options [8]. Gender bias also exists in the pattern of help seeking for mental health problems, and females are more likely to seek help from her primary health care physicians.

Many migrants in Western countries suffer from social and economic inequity that may adversely impact their mental health and well being. The number of international migrants worldwide is growing each year, reaching 244 million in 2015 [9]. Although limited research has been performed in this field, black, Asian and ethnic minorities are considered at increased risk of poor mental health. Depression and PTSD were more prevalent among immigrant black women within the UK and this association was related to the higher levels of sexual assaults they experience [10].

Refugees, asylum-seekers and stateless people are other groups at increased risk of mental health problems. In 2015, at least 65 million people were forcibly displaced worldwide, and they have higher rates of depression, PTSD and anxiety disorders. They have an increased vulnerability to mental health problems which may be linked to pre-migration experiences (exposure to war and trauma) and the post-migration situation refugees face (social isolation, separation from family, unemployment, inadequate housing and detention or difficulties with asylum procedures) [10]. More than 80% of the 50 million people affected by violent conflicts, civil wars and displacement are women and children [11]. Around one third of trafficked boys and girls have experienced physical or sexual violence. More than half of young trafficked survivors screened positive for depression, a third for anxiety disorders, at least 25% for PTSD, and 16% reported having suicidal thoughts [11].

People with lower intellectual ability have higher rates of common mental health disorders (25%) compared with people with average intellectual ability (17%). The prevalence of diagnosed mental health disorders in children with intellectual disability has been estimated in 36% compared to 8% among children without [10]. A UK survey found even a higher prevalence: 50% of mental health problems in individuals with learning disabilities [10].

People with physical disabilities and health problems are also at increased risk of poor mental health, in particular depression and anxiety. Chronic neurological conditions are associated with higher rates of mental health problems. More than one third of stroke survivors and 50% of patients suffering with Parkinson's disease have depression or anxiety [12, 13].

People who identify themselves as gay, lesbian, bisexual and/or transgender are also at higher risk of poor mental health, and they are two to three times more likely to report having a psychological problem compared to heterosexual people. In a 2011 UK survey, 1 in 7 gay and bisexual men had moderate to severe levels of mixed depression and anxiety, and 1 in 10 gay and bisexual men aged 16–19 had attempted to take their own lives [10].

People with multiple social disadvantages include offenders, substance misusing individuals and homeless population. 80% of homeless people in England reported having mental health issues and 45% were diagnosed as having a mental health condition [10]. Substance misuse (62%) was also common among the homeless population. A survey based in England found that 36% of prisoners had a disability or mental health problem, and 49% of women prisoners reported anxiety and depression compared with 23% of men [10]. Suicide rates within prisons are at least 4 times those of the general population. In USA, over half of the prison population has a serious mental illness [14].

2.2.3 Gender – Diagnosis and Prognosis

A consistent gender effect on the prevalence of common mental health disorders exists. Depression, anxiety, eating disorders, PTSD and somatoform disorders are more common in women whereas substance dependence, alcohol abuse, impulse control and antisocial personality disorders are more frequently observed in men [15].

Women have a higher lifetime prevalence of mood and anxiety disorders than men, and a later onset of psychoses such as schizophrenia. Data from a systematic review and meta-analysis from 1980–2013 found that women have higher rates of low mood (period prevalence: 7.3% vs 4%) and anxiety (8.7% vs 4.3%) [2]. Women also had higher lifetime prevalence rates for mood (14% vs 7.3%) and anxiety disorders (18.2% vs 10%) compared with men. The gender gap seems to be similar in developed countries, low-income and middle-income countries, although regional differences have been described.

Eating disorders affect 1.9% of women and 0.2% of men. The risk of developing PTSD after any traumatic event has been estimated in more than 20% for women and 8% for men. Lifetime prevalence for alcohol dependence is more than twice as high in men. In developed countries, 1 in 5 men and 1 in 12 women develop any degree of alcohol dependence during their life span [15].

Gender differences have also been reported on prevalence, risk factors, symptoms and course of mental health disorders. Women are more severely affected by poverty and are subjected to greater number of negative life events. Recognised risk factors for depression in women are summarised in Table 2.1.

Two gender-related course-moderating factors have also been noted: the incidence of completed suicide is higher in men, and mortality in depressed individuals is higher among depressed men. Suicide rates in men are double of those in women although women may present with more para-suicidal behaviours [15]. Men have also poorer physical health and respond more negatively to unemployment. Cultural issues related to masculinity may have a negative impact on mental health in men. Higher rates of suicide in men have been associated to male reluctance to express distress [15].

Table 2.1 Potential risk factors associated with gender effects and increased risk of depression in females

1. Biological factors
Genetic factors and gene-environment interactions
Sex hormone influences
Blunted hypothalamic-pituitary-adrenal axis response to stress in women
2. Individual psychological factors
Lower self esteem and dissatisfaction
Body shame and rumination
3. Psychosocial factors
Exposure and susceptibility to stressors
Experienced gender-based violence
– Childhood sexual abuse
– Domestic violence
– Sexual violence
4. Societal factors
Gender inequity
Discrimination in the workplace and professional career
Gender harassment

2.2.4   Life Span

Mental health problems occur across the life span. Exposure to adversity at a young age and adverse early life experiences are well known risk factors for mental disorders. A life course perspective is crucial to understand that vulnerability and exposure to harmful experiences and stress can be disruptive [16].

In England, around 10% of children and young people aged 5–16 had a clinically diagnosable mental health problem. Prevalence of common mental health disorders among this group was 4% for depression or anxiety, 6% for conduct disorder, 2% for hyperkinetic problems and 1% for autism and eating disorders [17].

Worldwide, between 10% and 20% of children and adolescents have mental disorders. Children living in poverty are five times at increased risk of mental illness [18]. A systematic review found a 2.5 times higher prevalence rate of depression and anxiety disorders among youths aged 10–15 from low socioeconomic status compared to those from higher status [19].

Prevalence of depression before puberty is low, and boys are more likely to meet criteria for major depression [15]. However the rate of depressive disorders during puberty up to age 18 doubles in girls. Then, from early adulthood to late in life, a higher prevalence for women appears and the female preponderance for depression continues into old age [15].

Women often play multiple roles in life (mothers, partners and carers) and may be working and running a household. They also have the responsibility for the care of family members and are exposed to more stressors. Pregnancy and puerperium are crucial stages in life in which women are at increased risk of mental health problems. Around 50% of women may suffer from transient low mood following delivery. One third of affective disorders detected after delivery were already present during pregnancy. Anxiety disorders increase in the perinatal period and quite often are undetected [20].

Mental health disorders become more prevalent in adulthood. The Marmot Review Team described some major risk factors for mental health in adult age including negative life events, poverty, low education, low economic status, unemployment and poor-quality employment [21].

Around 15% of people older than 60 suffer a mental disorder, mainly depression and dementia; anxiety disorders affect near 4% and substance abuse 1%. Elderly people are at higher risk of having depression, and associated risk factors are loss of status, poor physical health, chronic pain, reduction in social contacts, and bereavement. Depression in elderly women has been linked to social isolation and reduced contact with family. Indeed 10% of elderly people are socially isolated, and social isolation is a risk factor for poor mental health, poor cognition, alcohol dependence, suicidal ideation and death in the elderly [22].

The number of elderly people nowadays (900 million) is expected to rise to 2 billion in 2050. The rapid increase in population's age will increase age-related physical and mental health problems, as well as the risk of dementia. Caregiving for people with dementia is associated with significant psychological distress. High-levels of depression and anxiety have been found in caregivers of dementia patients, and dementia severity and lower support from other family members are predictive factors of depression in dementia caregivers [23].

2.2.5   Ethics

Bioethics in mental health is an emerging field. It has been proposed that bioethics should allude to vulnerable populations such as the mentally ill as an exception to a paradigm disproportionally emphasizing autonomy and informed consent. Traditional bioethics valued autonomy and its agent, informed consent. However, some criticism has risen as bioethics may have neglected ethic issues related to mental health in the past. Current reconsideration of bioethics includes the notions of agency, self-determination and present and future-selves [14].

Social inequality and stigmatization of psychiatric illness are also challenges for bioethics. Social inequalities are strongly associated to mental health inequalities. Mental health inequalities are *socially produced systematic differences in mental health between social groups that are avoidable and unjust*' [14]. Poverty, deprivation, unemployment and low education are associated with increased mental health problems [21]. Socioeconomically disadvantaged young people are two to three times more likely to develop mental health problems [10]. Between 35% and 50% of people with severe mental health problems in developed countries and more than three quarters in developing countries receive no treatment [24]. People suffering mental health problems are more likely to be victims of violence than those without. All these facts have important ethic implications that should be better addressed.

2.3   Discussion

There has been relatively little research about prevalence and risk factors of mental health disorders. Regional variation on estimates of common and severe mental health disorders exists. Variation in estimates seems to be greater for substance abuse. A gap in knowledge about prevalence in lower and middle income countries remains, and this fact affects mainly Asian and sub-Saharan countries where a lack of data exists.

From a cultural diversity and global perspective, the validity, reliability and cross-cultural adaptation of many mental health disorders diagnostic criteria remain problematic and this fact may affect the accuracy of data of epidemiological studies worldwide. There is a huge variation in DALYs attributed to mental health disorders across the world, and this fact requires further analysis. The inclusion of childhood disorders may be especially relevant for African countries in some of which up to 40% of the population are children.

WHO estimated in 2001 that one in four people would suffer a mental health condition at some point throughout their lives [25]. However, the most updated epidemiological data may not reflect the accuracy of the real burden of mental health problems [25]. Mental disorders are commonly under-diagnosed and only less than 50% of those meeting criteria for a common mental health problem are diagnosed or identified. In addition, many people do not have access to a mental health professional for diagnosis. For this reason, lifetime prevalence rates for mental problems may be higher than previously thought and could potentially affect even nearly half of the world's population.

Gender, ethnic and sexual minorities often have poor mental health. Cultural stigma, social inequality, discrimination and even lack of awareness about common mental health problems may explain poor mental health outcomes. Although some ethnic minority groups have a similar rate of mental health problems than white population, the consequences of mental illness in those minorities may be long lasting.

Gender is a social and cultural construct that has a deep impact on mental health risk, progression of illness, and also on socioeconomic status [26, 27]. Social determinants of health are also gender biased. Women are around 70% of the world's poor and earn significantly less than males when in paid work. Mental health research has frequently ignored gender differences, and the different risks and protective factors associated [28]. The cause of the gender gap is not well understood, and little research on gender effects has been done to explain this fact.

Domestic violence and sexual abuse are the strongest predictors of depression in adulthood. Sexual violence is a preventable risk factor to which women are exposed and is linked with high rates of PTSD, substance abuse, suicide attempts and medically unexplained symptoms. A gender effect is clearly identified, and lifetime prevalence rates of violence against women range from 16% to 50%, and nearly one in five women suffer rape or abuse in their lifetime. Domestic violence and abuse reflect social inequality between men and women [29]. Severity and duration of violence exposure are a significant predictive factor for mental health outcomes. Women who were exposed to childhood sexual abuse or physical partner violence in adult life have an increased four fold risk of having depression as adults [30].

Priority strategies that could prevent mental health problems in women include raising autonomy to exercise control in response to severe events; a better access to material resources that allow the possibility of making choices about women's own lives; and encouraging psychosocial support from family, friends and health providers [11].

Gender stereotypes such as "females are prone to emotional problems" and "men are prone to alcohol problems" may reinforce stigma and constraint help seeking patterns [26]. Gender differences in the pattern of help seeking, and the gender stereotypes in diagnosis may explain the reason why females are being prescribed more psychotropic drugs. In addition, women are more frequently diagnosed with depression than males, even when presenting with similar symptoms [11].

2.4 Conclusion

Mental and substance use disorders are the leading cause of disability worldwide. Furthermore, an increase in the burden of mental disease is expected in the next few decades. At least one out of every five young people will suffer at least one mental disorder through their lives. Children and adolescents exposed to neglect and substance abuse, women, elderly people and community groups suffering discrimination such as ethnic minorities, immigrants and refugees are at increased risk for mental disorders thorough their lifespan.

Women have a greater risk of depressive and anxiety disorders and men suffer a higher frequency of alcohol and substance use, antisocial behaviour and suicide. Social and environmental adversities may also have a major effect on the development of first depressive episodes through the life span, particularly in women. Mental health promotion policy should take into account the existence of a gender gap, and changes of socioeconomic trends that affect this gap should also be monitored.

Future Tasks
- An overview of epidemiology of mental health worldwide is difficult because prevalence studies are virtually absent in many low and middle income countries.
- Further epidemiological research including longitudinal studies across lifespan, the application of check list for risk factors and outcomes, and the analysis of comorbidities is needed.
- Prevalence studies should be based on community-representative samples rather than on selected clinical case-series studies. An interdisciplinary approach including biological and psychosocial factors is also encouraged.
- Research about violence-related health problems, specifically in women, is necessary as mental health issues have been poorly identified.
- The inclusion of gender aspects, cultural diversity and ethics in mental health should be considered desirable standards in the future.
- WHO advised that decreasing the depressed female overrepresentation could lessen the global burden caused by mental disorders. Health care providers require further training to successfully identify violent victimization. Policymakers should be aware of these facts.
- Additional monitoring about the impact of increased life expectancy and the greater prevalence of mental health disorders in the elderly is essential and more economic resources and involvement of policy makers is encouraged.
- Policies that reduce conflicts and stimulate actions to improve conditions of refugees and asylum-seekers may improve their mental health and decrease vulnerability.
- The WHO Mental Health Atlas may be a useful tool to track progress of these future pending tasks [31].

References

1. World Health Organization. (2011). *Global burden of mental disorders and the need for a comprehensive, coordinated response from health and social sectors at the country level: Report by the Secretariat.* Geneva: WHO. Available at: apps.who.int/gb/ebwha/pdf_files/EB130/B130_9-en.pdf. Accessed 15 Dec 2018.
2. Steel, Z., Marnane, C., Iranpour, C., Chey, T., Jackson, J. W., Patel, V., et al. (2014). The global prevalence of common mental disorders: A systematic review and meta-analysis 1980-2013. *International Journal of Epidemiology, 43*, 476–493.
3. Ferrari, A., Charlson, F., Norman, R., Patten, S. B., Freedman, G., Murray, C. J. L., et al. (2013). Burden of depressive disorders by country, sex, age, and year: Findings from the global burden of disease study 2010. *PLoS Medicine, 10*, 1–12.
4. Whiteford, H. A., Degenhardt, L., Rehm, J., Baxter, A. J., Ferrari, A. J., Erskine, H. E., et al. (2013). Global burden of disease attributable to mental and substance use disorders: Findings from the Global Burden of Disease Study 2010. *Lancet, 382*, 1575–1586.

5. Vos, T., Barber, R. M., Bell, B., Bertozzi-Villa, A., Biryukov, S., Bolliger, I., et al. (2013). Global, regional, and national incidence, prevalence, and years lived with disability for 301 acute and chronic diseases and injuries in 188 countries, 1990–2013: A systematic analysis for the Global Burden of Disease study. *The Lancet, 386*, 743–800.
6. Bachmann, S. (2018). Epidemiology of suicide and the psychiatric perspective. *International Journal of Environmental Research and Public Health, 15*(7).
7. Gopalkrishnan, N. (2015). Cultural diversity and mental health. *Australian Psychiatry, 23*, 6–8.
8. APA. (2013). *Diagnostic and statistical manual of mental disorders* (5th ed.). Washington, DC: American Psychiatric Association.
9. United Nations. *Department of Economic and Social Affairs, Population Division. International Migration Report 2015: Highlights*. New York: United Nations, 2016.
10. Mental Health Foundation. (2016). *Fundamental facts about mental health 2016*. London: Mental Health Foundation. Available at: https://www.mentalhealth.org.uk/publications/funda-mental-facts-about-mental-health-2016. Accessed 20 Dec 2018.
11. World Health Organization. (2018). *Gender and women's health*. Geneva: WHO. Available at: https://www.who.int/mental_health/prevention/genderwomen/en. Accessed 20 Dec 2018.
12. Carod Artal, F. J., Ferreira Coral, L., Trizotto, D. S., & Menezes Moreira, C. (2009). Poststroke depression: Prevalence and determinants in Brazilian stroke patients. *Cerebrovascular Diseases, 28*, 157–165.
13. Carod-Artal, F. J., Ziomkowski, S., Mourão Mesquita, H., & Martínez-Martin, P. (2008). Anxiety and depression: Main determinants of health-related quality of life in Brazilian patients with Parkinson's disease. *Parkinsonism & Related Disorders, 14*, 102–108.
14. Williams, A. R. (2016). Opportunities in reform: Bioethics and mental health ethics. *Bioethics, 30*, 221–226.
15. Kuehner, C. (2017). Why is depression more common among women than among men? *Lancet Psychiatry, 4*, 146–158.
16. Carod-Artal, F. J. (2017). Social determinants of mental health. In S. Bährer-Kohler & F. Carod-Artal (Eds.), *Global mental health* (pp. 33–46). London: Springer.
17. Department of Health and the Scottish Executive. (2004). *Mental health of children and young people in Great Britain*. Available at: www.hscic.gov.uk/catalogue/PUB06116/ment-heal-chil-youn-peop-gb-2004-rep1.pdf. Accessed 15 Dec 2018.
18. World Health Organization. (2014). *Mental health: A state of well being*. Geneva: WHO. Available at: http://www.who.int/features/factfiles/mental_health/mental_health_facts/en/. Accessed 15 Dec 2018.
19. Lemstra, M., Neudorf, C., D'Arcy, C., Kunst, A., Warren, L. M., & Bennett, N. R. (2008). A systematic review of depressed mood and anxiety by SES in youth aged 10–15 years. *Canadian Journal of Public Health, 99*, 125–129.
20. Howard, L. M., Molyneaux, E., Dennis, C. L., Rochat, T., Stein, A., & Milgrom, J. (2014). Non-psychotic mental disorders in the perinatal period. *Lancet, 384*, 1775–1788.
21. Marmot Review Team. (2010). *Fair society, healthy lives: Strategic review of health inequalities in England post-2010*. London: Marmot Review. Available at: http://www.instituteofhealthequity.org. Accessed 20 Dec 2018.
22. Grundy, E., van Campen, C., Deeg, D., Dourgnon, P., Huisman, M., Ploubidis, G., et al. (2013). *Health inequalities and the health divide among older people in the WHO European region: The European review on the social determinants of health and the health divide (report of the task group on older people)*. Copenhagen: World Health Organization Regional Office for Europe.
23. Omranifard, V., Haghighizadeh, E., & Akouchekian, S. (2018). Depression in main caregivers of dementia patients: Prevalence and predictors. *Advanced Biomedical Research, 7*, 34.
24. Demyttenaere, K., Bruffaerts, R., Posada-Villa, J., Gasquet, I., Kovess, V., Lepine, J. P., et al. (2004). Prevalence, severity, and unmet need for treatment of mental disorders in the World Health Organization World Mental Health Surveys. *JAMA, 292*, 2581–2590.

25. World Health Organization. *Mental disorders affect one in four people*. Available at: https://www.who.int/whr/2001/media_centre/press_release/en/. Accessed 15 Dec 2018.
26. World Health Organization. (2000). *Gender disparities in mental health*. Geneva: WHO Department of Mental Health and Substance Abuse.
27. Riecher Rossler, A. (2017). Sex and gender differences in mental disorders. *Lancet Psychiatry, 4*, 8–9.
28. Howard, L., Ehrlich, A., Gamlen, F., & Oram, S. (2017). Gender-neutral mental health research is sex and gender biased. *Lancet Psychiatry, 4*, 9–11.
29. Oram, S., Khalifeh, H., & Howard, L. (2017). Violence against women and mental health. *Lancet Psychiatry, 4*, 159–170.
30. Gallo, E. A. G., Munhoz, T. N., Loret de Mola, C., & Murray, J. (2018). Gender differences in the effects of childhood maltreatment on adult depression and anxiety: A systematic review and meta-analysis. *Child Abuse & Neglect, 79*, 107–114.
31. World Health Organization. (2018). *Mental health atlas 2017*. Geneva: WHO. Available at: http://apps.who.int/iris/bitstream/handle/10665/272735/9789241514019-eng.pdf. Accessed 13 Jan 2019.

Chapter 3
Aspects of Diversity and Lifespan

Sabine Bährer-Kohler

Key Points
- Wellner [34] conceptualized diversity as representing a multitude of individual differences, characteristics, specifications and similarities that exist among people [33, p. 3].
- Diversity can be along the dimensions of race, ethnicity, gender, sexual orientation, social class, socio-economic status, age, physical abilities, educational background, and family status and structures [23].
- Stages in the lifespan of the members of the human family such as pregnancy, childhood, adolescence and adult age are characterized by several and diverse components, influenced by national, transnational and global factors, characteristics, differences and similarities.
- All the lifespan stages are interrelated to mental health aspects and vice versa.
- All Sustainable Development Goals (SDGs) of the United Nations should be implemented in all presentations and actions for respectively about diversity and lifespan [30]. SDGs address the global challenges, including those related to poverty, inequality, environmental degradation, prosperity, peace and justice [31], and achieve a better and more sustainable future for all.
- More sound scientific studies/ publications related to diversity and lifespan are required, especially more meta-analysis. Solid and wide-ranging scientific data are limited in several countries.

(continued)

S. Bährer-Kohler (✉)
Dr. Bährer-Kohler & Partner, Basel, Switzerland

International University of Catalonia (UIC), Barcelona, Spain
e-mail: sabine.baehrer@datacomm.ch

© The Author(s) 2019
S. Bährer-Kohler, B. Bolea-Alamanac (eds.), *Diversity in Global Mental Health*,
SpringerBriefs in Psychology, https://doi.org/10.1007/978-3-030-29112-9_3

- Scientific results can document data and effects of diversity aspects and lifespan, the effects and consequences should be named and analyzed, negative effects should be reduced or eliminated, and problems and crisis situations minimized or solved with the aid and support of national and global federations, associations, governments, institutions, stakeholders, heads of states and others.
- All members of the human family [28] are at the core when relating to aspects of diversity and lifespan.

3.1   Introduction

The term lifespan refers to the maximum number of years that a human lives. Japan's average life expectancy at birth is still the highest in the world, approximately 83.7 years according to the World Health Statistics report [37] released by WHO in May 2017 [38]. This average, however, shows clear gender differences, with approximately 6 years difference in life expectancy at birth between women and men [38].

The World Health Statistics 2017, documents different distributions of death (2005–2015) assigned to different age groups of males and females. Additionally, a new study by [8] shows, with restrictions, that current results strongly suggest that the maximum lifespan of humans is more or less fixed and subject to natural constraints. Lifespan stages are characterized and influenced by several components, such as diversity, health components, social determinants [39], psychosocial developments [9], motivational components [13], active and goal-oriented roles ([16] in [13]), coping ([5] in [13]), and, for example, political and economic factors, environmental, national and global circumstances.

The definition of diversity differs from person to person, from organization to organization, from publication to publication [33].

Wellner [34] conceptualized diversity as representing a multitude of individual differences, characteristics and similarities that exist among people [33].

Diversity can be along the dimensions of race, ethnicity, gender, sexual orientation, social class, socio-economic status, age, physical abilities, educational background, and family status [23].

3.2   Content

"Whereas recognition of the inherent dignity and of the equal and inalienable rights of all members of the human family is the foundation of freedom, justice and peace in the world." Universal Declaration of Human Rights, Preamble [28].

Lifespan stages of the members of the human family such as pregnancy, childhood, adolescence and adult age are characterized by several and diverse components, influenced by national and global factors, characteristics, differences and similarities. General socioeconomic, cultural, political and environmental conditions, social and community networks and individual factors characterize these stages [7]. All lifespan stages are a process, not a status; all processes need adaptation, development and protection.

Pregnancy is a period of life that is an individual challenge for each woman; it can be an amazing and glorious time. Women are individuals, with individual characteristics, from a biomedical point of view and, for example, from a psychological point of view. However, pregnancies around the globe have similarities; roughly over 135 million women give birth per year [45].

Nevertheless, women live in different settings, cultural and political settings, family networks, social class and societal situations. Health systems are differently structured, with different services and access to services.

Childhood Each child is an individual, lives in individual settings, cultural settings, family structures, social classes, social and environmental settings. Each country, each region has specific regulations and/or services for children, different social and health systems and access to health care for children [46]. In addition, different school systems, access to the school systems, different training and educational options. There are similarities between all children around the globe, but as well, there are great differences around the globe, gender related [27].

Adolescence is a period characterized by a specific age group, i.e. persons aged between 10 and 19. It is a period with a great number of changes and challenges. Adolescents have to face and react to specific tasks, find their own ways regarding space, voice, audience, influence; they have to find and build up their own roles in their specific settings, cultural settings, circumstances and social and political networks [47]. It is a process of maturation, and not always untroubled. It is a process embedded, for example, in health-, social-, gender and racial aspects. There are similarities and great differences around the globe.

Adult age is a period for each individual, with biological adulthood and non-biological adulthood [49]. But age alone does not an adult make. Characterized is this period, for example, by the responsibility of and for one's own life, specific rights, working conditions, living conditions, and own parenthood. Adult age has similarities around the globe and great differences. These are related to different settings, cultural conditions, social conditions, family networks, social class, gender, socioeconomic and economic factors, societal and political situations, and many other conditions.

Old age is a period with biological adaptations, with reductions and with chronological, biological, psychological and social changes and challenges [29]. It is related to perceptions, cultural settings, and possibilities or opportunities. Different settings, family networks, social class and societal situations have a great input and influence, especially for the palliative care settings. Health systems and social care systems for old age and the oldest old are differently structured around the globe, sometimes unexciting, sometimes with different service supplies, different access to services and different ways to finance it. Healthy ageing differs; the participation of elderly people differs around the globe.

In the following, the focus area of pregnancy will be presented in more detail.

3.2.1   Lifespan – Diversity – Pregnancy Aspects

The social determinants of health (SDH) are the conditions in which people are born, grow, work, live, and age: the conditions that influence health [39]. These conditions influence a pregnancy.

The World Health Organization underlined in 2016 that pregnancy-related deaths and diseases remain unacceptably high. In 2015, an estimated 303,000 women died from pregnancy- or delivery- related complications, 2.7 million babies died during their first 28 days of life and 2.6 million babies were stillborn [36].

Developing and developed countries: Approximately 99% of all maternal deaths occur in developing countries [40]. Globally in 2015, births in the richest 20 per cent of households were more than twice as likely to be attended by skilled health professionals than those in the poorest 20 per cent of households (89 per cent versus 43 per cent) [40]. Skilled health professionals are professionals educated, trained and regulated to national and international standards [42, p. 2, box 3].

Birth in private facilities: A current analysis [22], with data across countries and over time in Cambodia, India, Indonesia, the Philippines, Bangladesh and Nepal, documents that there is an increase in the use of facilities for birth, and an increase in the use of private facilities.

Rural areas: Maternal mortality is clearly higher in women living in rural areas, and among poorer communities [40]. This is related to many components. For example, rural women have less access to health care than urban women [1]. In addition, the access to health care for rural residents is often complicated, (a) by patient factors and (b) by the delivery of care [1]. Here, traveling long distances is only one reason [12].

Single-parent families: Single-parent families are documented to be increasing around the world [14]. Approximately 15 per cent of children worldwide live in single-parent families, and most of these households are headed by women.

Average age of women giving birth: In most of the OECD countries, the average age at which women give birth now stands around 30 years or above [19, p. 1]. Nevertheless, more than approximately one-third of women in developing countries give birth before the age of 20 years ([24] in [4]).

3.2.2 Adolescent Pregnancy

Age/regions/adolescent pregnancy: Adolescent pregnancies are a global problem that occurs either in high, as well as in middle and low income countries [43], but adolescent pregnancies are more likely to occur in marginalized communities [43].

About 252 million adolescent girls aged 15–19 live in developing regions of the world [21]. Approximately 16 million girls aged 15–19 and approximately 2.5 million girls under 16 give birth each year in developing regions [43]. Latin America with the Caribbean continues to be the region of the world with the second highest adolescent pregnancy rate world-wide [21]. The global adolescent pregnancy rate is roughly 46 births per 1000 girls, while adolescent pregnancy rates in Latin America and the Caribbean are estimated at 66.5 births per 1000 girls aged 15–19, second only to Sub-Saharan Africa [21]. Other data by the UNFPA, the United Nations sexual and reproductive health agency, show that every single day in developing countries some 20,000 girls under 18 give birth [26].

Social determinants/adolescent pregnancy: Maness and Buhi [17] have documented and related to social determinants of health (SDH) and pregnancy of adolescent girls that

- poverty and
- family structures were the areas most often represented.

UNFPA [26] added that early pregnancy is often a consequence of

- little or no access to school,
- little or no information, or
- little or no health care.

Effects of early pregnancy:
- Adolescent pregnancy often takes an enormous toll on a girl's education, training, and income-earning potential [26].
- Many adolescents are not yet physically and psychologically ready for pregnancy or childbirth, and are therefore more vulnerable to complications [26]. In addition, the World Health Organization underlined that young adolescents face a much higher risk of complications and death as a result of pregnancy than others, i.e. older women [40]. A current study in Korea documents differences in detail between teenagers with other age groups during pregnancy. Lee et al. [15] underlined that teenage mothers are at a high risk for maternal and neonatal complications. For example, teenage mothers were more likely to have an abortion (33.4%) than to deliver a baby when compared with other age groups.
- The current leading cause of death for 15 to 19-year-old girls globally is complications during pregnancy and childbirth [44].

Aspects of ethnic groups: Ethnic aspects influence pregnancy, birth, and maternal death. Women belonging to specific ethnic groups characterized by small body size often have less weight during pregnancy [20]. Further disparities can also be documented in maternal mortality rates. For example, the estimated white British maternal death rate is 8 per 100,000 maternities, compared to approximately 28 for the Black ethnic group (combined) and approximately 33 for Black Africans [10]. Despite limited specific, high-quality evidence, there is consistent data of maternal death among ethnic minority women that suggest that black and ethnic minority women do not access or receive optimal care and that this can increase their risk of morbidity and death [3, p. 181]. Many factors are found to be associated with the higher mortality among black and ethnic minority women, who are often in marginalized groups, including:

- domestic violence or other types of abuse,
- communication and transaction problems,
- refugee and recent immigration status,
- poor and limited access to care and/or information about it,
- substandard care provision.

Global Mental Health Aspects: For many women, pregnancy increases their vulnerability to psychiatric conditions or mental diseases. But pregnancy during adolescence is a risk factor for adverse psychosocial outcomes, including psychiatric symptoms and disorders [25]. Here, pregnant teens appear to have a high rate of mental health problems in many and different ways ([18] in [48]).

Current scientific data suggests demonstrably that pregnant and parenting adolescents run a greater risk of experiencing depressive symptoms than pregnant and postpartum adult women [25].

In Brazil, teenagers reported a relative high prevalence (32.5%) of psychiatric illness during the 12 months preceding the birth of their child, including substance-use disorders, psychotic disorders and anxiety disorders (15.7%), as well as post-traumatic stress disorder (PTSD), and eating disorders, or with severe disturbances of a person's eating behavior ([18] in [48]).

Worldwide, approximately 10% of pregnant women and 13% of women who have just given birth experience some mental disorder, primarily depression [41]. In developing countries, this figure is even higher, i.e. 15.6% experience a mental disorder during pregnancy and approximately 19.8% after childbirth [35]. Moreover, a current meta-analysis confirmed the data and showed that about 20% of mothers in developing countries experience clinical depression after childbirth [41].

Childbearing years are a time of increased vulnerability to the onset or recurrence of major depressive disorders, thus placing particularly young women at the risk of suffering from severe affective impairment during pregnancy [11].

In severe cases, the mothers' suffering can be so severe that they may even commit or attempt suicide [41]. These statements are in line with other epidemiological

data, which has demonstrated that suicidal ideation is a relatively frequent compli-
cation of pregnancy in both developed and developing countries [11] and particularly in pregnant adolescents [6].

3.3 Discussion

To discuss aspects of diversity and lifespan means discussing an unending topic. It
is not possible to conclude or to summarize all the aspects and facts in this field.
Many aspects of diversity influence in both ways. However, it is possible to present
detailed aspects, relationships and effects on specific issues and topics, as in and for
many other scientific areas.

Any stage in life is a process, not a status. In addition, interdependencies, depen-
dencies and restrictions are documentable in this process.

For example:

- If a young adolescent has to marry because the family has decided so, many
  individual processes and developments of the young adolescent will be not
  possible.
- If palliative care services do not exist in a country or in a region of a country, a
  person and his/her family are unable to decide about specific palliative care
  issues.
- Self-management of diversity aspects will be unsuccessful or limited if the relevant framework and conditions do not exist.

The basis of all development is rights, human rights, protection and support. But
they have to be implemented, for example, by laws and regulations in societies,
families, and individuals.

Reality, however, faces other situations, events and conditions, all over the globe.
The world is suffering from a very bad case of "trust deficit disorder", warned UN
chief Antonio Guterres at the end of September 2018 in New York ([32]).

Awareness of issues is the starter, motivation is the pusher, and the results are the
benefits. It is a long-lasting process demanding enormous engagement from many,
if not from "all" the parties involved. This demands the ability to reflect, to create,
to investigate and to permit development. However, development and processes call
for views, leadership, sustainability and structures. International development and
processes in specific areas need international institutions, international bodies like
the United Nations. If these institutions cannot support or eradicate critical or urgent
aspects related to diversity and lifespan, further development will be restricted or
limited.

Race, ethnicity, gender and social class have, like many other diversity aspects, a
huge radius and influence, but they also offer empowerment, chances, opportunities
and possibilities.

3.4 Remarks & Conclusion

- Stages in the lifespan are characterized and influenced by several components, all over the globe, for example by diversity aspects, health components, and social determinants [39].
- Diversity is a widespread dimension with many facets and aspects.
- Scientific results can document data and effects of diversity aspects and lifespan; the effects and consequences should be named and analyzed; negative effects should be reduced or eradicated and problems or critical situations minimized or solved with the support of national and global federations, associations, institutions, stakeholders, governments, heads of states and others.
- All the stages in a lifespan are interrelated to mental health aspects and vice versa [2].
- The basis for further development is human rights, protections, laws, regulations and the awareness of individuals, societies, international leaders, stakeholders, and decision makers.
- Always required are sound, sustainable, scientific publications and documentations.

Future Tasks
- More scientific studies/publications related to diversity and lifespan are needed, especially more meta-analysis. Sound and wide-ranging scientific data are scarce in several countries.
- More scientific studies/publications related to global mental health and diversity throughout the lifespan are required.
- The term "diversity" has to be defined in a global dimension and in great detail.
- Awareness of diversity, lifespan and mental health in a global context is needed.
- The leading people, decision makers and chairpersons should use national and international networks and expert experiences to reduce adolescent pregnancy, as one example of many in this context.
- All Sustainable Development Goals (SDGs) of the United Nations should be implemented in all presentations about diversity and lifespan [30].
- Far more visions, activities, and engagement are required to achieve a better and more sustainable future for all [31] and to avoid further "trust deficit disorders".
- So as to "crack hard nuts" during a process it needs, for example, the will to do it, energy, courage and, always, sound scientific information and publications.

References

1. ACOG- American College of Obstetricians and Gynecologists. (2014). *Committee on Health Care for Underserved Women*. Health Disparities in Rural Women. https://www.acog.org/Clinical-Guidance-and-Publications/Committee-Opinions/Committee-on-Health-Care-for-Underserved-Women/Health-Disparities-in-Rural-Women. Retrieved 24 Aug 2018.
2. Aktionsbündnis Seelische Gesundheit. (2018). *Psychische Erkrankungen*. https://www.seelischegesundheit.net/themen/psychische-erkrankungen. Retrieved 1 Oct 2018.
3. Ameh, C. A., & van den Broek, N. (2008). Clinical governance. Increased risk of maternal death among ethnic minority women in the UK. *The Obstetrician & Gynaecologist, 10*, 177–182. https://obgyn.onlinelibrary.wiley.com/doi/pdf/10.1576/toag.10.3.177.27421. Retrieved 20 Sept 2018.
4. Ayyuba, R., Sayyid, A., Takai, I. U., et al. (2016). Age at first pregnancy among primigravidae attending antenatal clinic at a Tertiary Hospital in Kano. *Archives of International Surgery, 6*(2), 111–114. http://www.archintsurg.org/article.asp?issn=2278-9596;year=2016;volume=6;issue=2;spage=111;epage=114;aulast=Ayyuba;type=0. Retrieved 25 Sept 2018.
5. Boerner, K. (2004). Adaptation to disability among middle-aged and older adults: The role of assimilative and accommodative coping. *Journal of Gerontology Series B: Psychological Sciences and Social Sciences., 59*, 35–42.
6. Da Cunha Coelho, F. M., Pinheiro, R. T., Silva, R. A., et al. (2013). Major depressive disorder during teenage pregnancy: Socio-demographic, obstetric and psychosocial correlates. *Revista Brasileira de Psiquiatria, 35*(1). São Paulo. http://www.scielo.br/scielo.php?script=sci_arttext&pid=S1516-44462013000100009. Retrieved 20 Sept 2018.
7. Dahlgren, G., & Whitehead, M. (1991). *The Dahlgren-Whitehead model*. Stockholm, Sweden: Institute for Futures Studies.
8. Dong, X., Milholland, B., & Vijg, J. (2016). Evidence for a limit to human lifespan. *Nature, 538*, 257–259. https://www.nature.com/articles/nature19793. Retrieved 21 Aug 2018.
9. Erikson, E. H. (1959). *Identity and the life cycle*. New York: International Universities Press.
10. Garcia, R., Ali, N., Papadopoulos, C., & Randhawa, G. (2015). Specific antenatal interventions for Black, Asian and Minority Ethnic (BAME) pregnant women at high risk of poor birth outcomes in the United Kingdom: A scoping review. *BMC Pregnancy and Childbirth, 15*, 22. https://bmcpregnancychildbirth.biomedcentral.com/articles/10.1186/s12884-015-0657-2. Retrieved 20 Sept 2018.
11. Gentile, S. (2011). Suicidal mothers. *Journal of Injury and Violence Research, 3*(2), 90–97. https://www.ncbi.nlm.nih.gov/pmc/articles/PMC3134924/. Retrieved 27 Sept 2018.
12. Graves, L. (2012). New approaches for rural maternity care. *Canadian Family Physician, 58*(10), 1067–1068. https://www.ncbi.nlm.nih.gov/pmc/articles/PMC3470492/. Retrieved 20 Sept 2018.
13. Heckhausen, J., Wrosch, C., & Schulz, R. (2010). A motivational theory of life-span development. *Psychological Review, 117*(1), 32–60. https://www.ncbi.nlm.nih.gov/pmc/articles/PMC2820305/#R120. Retrieved 22 Aug 2018.
14. Kim, J.-E., Lee, J. Y., & Lee, S. H. (2018). Single mothers' experiences with pregnancy and child rearing in Korea: Discrepancy between social services/policies and single mothers' needs. *International Journal of Environmental Research and Public Health, 15*(5), 955.
15. Lee, S. H., Lee, S. M., Lim, N. G., et al. (2016). Differences in pregnancy outcomes, prenatal care utilization, and maternal complications between teenagers and adult women in Korea. *Medicine (Baltimore), 95*(34), e4630. https://www.ncbi.nlm.nih.gov/pmc/articles/PMC5400327/. Retrieved 23 Aug 2018.
16. Lerner, R. M. (2001). *Concepts and theories of human development* (3rd ed.). Psychology Press; In Heckhausen et al. 2010.

17. Maness, S. B., & Buhi, E. R. (2016). Associations between social determinants of health and pregnancy among young people: A systematic review of research published during the past 25 years. *Public Health Reports, 131*(1), 86–99. https://www.ncbi.nlm.nih.gov/pmc/articles/PMC4716476/. Retrieved 22 Aug 2018.
18. Mitsuhiro, S. S., Chalem, E., Barros, M. C. M., Guinsburg, R., & Laranjeira, R. (2009). Brief report: Prevalence of psychiatric disorders in pregnant teenagers. *Journal of Adolescence, 32*, 747–752.
19. OECD. (2018). *OECD Family Database.* http://www.oecd.org/els/family/database.htm. Retrieved 25 Sept 2018.
20. Ota, E., Haruna, M., Suzuki, M., et al. (2011). Maternal body mass index and gestational weight gain and their association with perinatal outcomes in Viet Nam. *Bulletin of the World Health Organization, 89*, 127–136. http://www.who.int/bulletin/volumes/89/2/10-077982/en/. Retrieved 24 Aug 2018.
21. PAHO- Pan American Health Organization. (2018). *Latin America and the Caribbean have the second highest adolescent pregnancy rates in the world.* https://www.paho.org/hq/index.php?option=com_content&view=article&id=14163%3Alatin-america-and-the-caribbean-have-the-second-highest-adolescent-pregnancy-rates-in-the-world&catid=740%3Apress-releases&Itemid=1926&lang=pt. Retrieved 24 Aug 2018.
22. Pomeroy, A. M., Koblinsky, M., & Alva, S. (2014). Who gives birth in private facilities in Asia? A look at six countries. *Health Policy and Planning, 29*(1), 38–i47. https://academic.oup.com/heapol/article/29/suppl_1/i38/637255. Retrieved 25 Sept 2018.
23. Queensborough Community College (2018). *Definition of diversity.* http://www.qcc.cuny.edu/diversity/definition.html. Retrieved 22 Aug 2018.
24. Rabbi, A. M., & Kabir, M. H. (2013). Factors influencing age at first birth of Bangladeshi women- a multivariate approach. *American Journal of Public Health Research, 1*, 191–195.
25. Siegel, R. S., & Brandon, A. R. (2014). Adolescents, pregnancy, and mental health. *Journal of Pediatric and Adolescent Gynecology, 27*(3), 138–150. https://www.ncbi.nlm.nih.gov/pubmed/24559618. Retrieved 20 Sept 2018.
26. UNFPA- United Nations Population Fund. (2018). *Adolescent pregnancy.* https://www.unfpa.org/adolescent-pregnancy. Retrieved 20 Sept 2018.
27. UNICEF- United Nations International Children's Emergency Fund. (2018). *For every child.* https://www.unicef.org/. Retrieved 25 Sept 2018.
28. UN- United Nations. (1948). *The Universal Declaration of Human Rights (UDHR).* http://www.un.org/en/universal-declaration-human-rights/. Retrieved 25 Sept 2018.
29. UN- United Nations. (2018). *Ageing.* http://www.un.org/en/sections/issues-depth/ageing/. Retrieved 25 Sept 2018.
30. UN- United Nations. (2018). *Sustainable development. Knowledge platform.* https://sustainabledevelopment.un.org/. Retrieved 26 Sept 2018.
31. UN- United Nations. (2018). *About the sustainable development goals.* https://www.un.org/sustainabledevelopment/sustainable-development-goals/. Retrieved 27 Sept 2018.
32. United Nations/UN Secretary General. (2018). *Secretary-general's address to the general assembly.* https://www.un.org/sg/en/content/sg/statement/2018-09-25/secretary-generals-address-general-assembly-delivered-trilingual. Retrieved 23 Jan 2019.
33. Washington, D. (2008). *The concept of diversity.* http://dwashingtonllc.com/images/pdf/publications/the_concept_of_diversity.pdf. Retrieved 22 Aug 2018.
34. Wellner, A. (2000). How do you spell diversity? *Training, 37*(4).
35. WHO- World Health Organization. (2014). *Mental health: A state of well-being.* Geneva: World Health Organization. URL: http://www.who.int/features/factfiles/mental_health/en/. Retrieved 24 Nov 2014.
36. WHO- World Health Organization. (2016). *New guidelines on antenatal care for a positive pregnancy experience.* http://www.who.int/reproductivehealth/news/antenatal-care/en/. Retrieved 23 Aug 2018.

37. WHO- World Health Organization. (2017). *World Health Statistics 2017: Monitoring health for the SDGs*. http://www.who.int/gho/publications/world_health_statistics/2017/EN_WHS2017_TOC.pdf; http://apps.who.int/iris/bitstream/handle/10665/255336/9789241565486-eng.pdf;jsessionid=372E2696645F5E9AC37169302902BEE2?sequence=1. Retrieved 21 Aug 2018.
38. WHO- World Health Organization. (2018). *Japan has the highest life expectancy- the World Health Statistics 2017 report*. http://www.who.int/kobe_centre/mediacentre/whs/en/. Retrieved 22 Aug 2018.
39. WHO- World Health Organization. (2018). *What are social determinants of health?* http://www.who.int/social_determinants/en/. Retrieved 22 Aug 2018.
40. WHO- World Health Organization. (2018). *Maternal mortality*. http://www.who.int/en/news-room/fact-sheets/detail/maternal-mortality. Retrieved 23 Aug 2018.
41. WHO- World Health Organization. (2018). *Maternal mental health*. http://www.who.int/mental_health/maternal-child/maternal_mental_health/en/. Retrieved 24 Aug 2018.
42. WHO- World Health Organization. (2018). *Definition of skilled health personnel providing care during childbirth: The 2018 joint statement by WHO, UNFPA, UNICEF, ICM, ICN, FIGO and IPA*. http://apps.who.int/iris/bitstream/handle/10665/272818/WHO-RHR-18.14-eng.pdf?ua=1. Retieved 20 Sept 2018).
43. WHO. (2018). *Adolescent pregnancy. Key facts*. http://www.who.int/news-room/fact-sheets/detail/adolescent-pregnancy. Retrieved 20 Sept 2018.
44. WHO. (2018). *Adolescents: Health risks and solutions. Key facts*. http://www.who.int/en/news-room/fact-sheets/detail/adolescents-health-risks-and-solutions. Retrieved 20 Sept 2018).
45. WHO. (2018). *10 facts on maternal health*. http://www.who.int/features/factfiles/maternal_health/maternal_health_facts/en/index2.html. Retrieved 25 Sept 2018.
46. WHO. (2018). *Child health*. http://www.who.int/topics/child_health/en/. Retrieved 25 Sept 2018.
47. WHO. (2018). *How young people can engage in global health and development*. http://www.who.int/health-topics/adolescents/coming-of-age-adolescent-health/adolescence%2D%2D-global-health-development. Retrieved 25 Sept 2018.
48. Weis, J. R., & Greene, J. A. (2016). Mental health in pregnant adolescents: Focus on psychopharmacology. *Journal of Pediatrics, 169*, 297–304.
49. World Bank Group. (2018). *Population ages 15–64 (% of total)*. https://data.worldbank.org/indicator/SP.POP.1564.TO.ZS?view=chart. Retrieved 25 Sept 2018.

Chapter 4
Women and Gender, Diversity and Mental Health

Chonnakarn Jatchavala and Pichet Udomratn

Key Points
- Gender is a determinant of mental health [1].
- Differences in gender and sexual orientation are accepted as a part of the spectrum of human condition [2]
- Emerging gender identities involve an interplay of bio- psycho-social factors and culture [2]
- Sex specific mental disorders exist such as premenstrual dysphoric disorder (PMDD)
- Violence against women, including sexual violence, causes severe emotional distress, and is rarely disclosed by the victims [3].
- Mental health providers should focus on providing women with resources to enable them to overcome such traumatic events, and encourage them to exercise their autonomy for making their own choices, in response to these severe life events [3]
- "A life-course perspective" is a beneficial framework for promoting the health needs of all genders, and to understand individuals considering their own experiences and social and cultural context (For example: family, peers, work setting) [4]
- Transgender identities should have access to gender affirmation, with appropriate health care services [5]
- Clinical assessment of gender identity, gender perception and gender expression; should be conducted in a setting of collaborative care using a multidisciplinary approach [6]
- Health care providers have a significant role promoting best practices on individual emotional and physical health needs, for the care of every gender, regardless of their specific identities and expressions [6]
- Social stigma and negative experiences from gender-based discrimination [7] are the most frequently occurring concerns in trans-gender people.

(continued)

C. Jatchavala (✉) · P. Udomratn
Prince of Songkla University, Department of Psychiatry, Songkhla, Thailand

© The Author(s) 2019
S. Bährer-Kohler, B. Bolea-Alamanac (eds.), *Diversity in Global Mental Health*,
SpringerBriefs in Psychology, https://doi.org/10.1007/978-3-030-29112-9_4

- To protect against gender-based harassment, victimization and stigmatization; stake holders, such as: general practitioners, pediatricians, mental health providers, educators and school administrators should promote, and enforce policies against-bullying [8].
- Federal governments should prioritize laws against gender discrimination and gender-based violence, by offering equal employment opportunities, regardless of gender identity and expression [8].

4.1 Introduction

The World Health Organization has declared gender as a critical determinant of mental health and recognized that social and cultural factors such as discrimination can contribute to psychiatric illness [1]. Specific mental health difficulties reported by women have been under-recognized by health providers, such as post-partum depression and premenstrual dysphoric disorder (PMDD) [9]. Similar issues arise within the LGBTQ population. Neglect secondary to stigma, social discrimination and lack of access to appropriate mental health services may explain the increased suicide rate in this population [7]. Although gender diversity issues have progressively become more acceptable, and more acknowledged, many health providers are faced with inadequate clinical education in order to clarify these important concepts we provide the following definitions [6]

- *Gender identity* is a deep, internal sense of being male, female, a combination of both or in between [6] (non-binary) or neither (gender neutral).
- *Gender expression* is the external way to express gender, such as clothes [6].
- *Gender perception* is the way other people understand an individual's gender expression [6]
- *Sexual orientation* is gender identity, regarding gender(s) to which they are sexually attracted [6]

This chapter aims to conceptualize as well as appraise mental health evidence regarding women and gender diversity. The authors also expect to fill the gaps of knowledge in this area to promote mental health.

4.2 Content

4.2.1 Women, Diversity and Mental Health

4.2.1.1 Mental Illnesses and Risk Factors Affecting Women Specifically

The World Health Organization considers women's mental health an essential concern. Women have higher rates of common mental disorders (CMD) [1]. A survey from the National Health Service (NHS) found that, overall, CMD's were diagnosed in one in five women, and women aged 16–24 years of age were reported as having about three times more common psychiatric symptoms, compared with men of the same age [10]. Self-harm rates have also greatly increased, among young women from; 4% in 2000 to 19.7% in 2014, depressive disorders will become the second leading cause of years living with a disability by 2020 globally [1, 11].

Unipolar depression is stated as having a 1.6-fold greater incidence in women, however; this difference reduces with age [12]. The interplay of biological, racial/ethnic-related, socio-cultural, nutritional, educational and other socio-economic factors are considered root causes of most mental illnesses [13, 14], but women's depression is believed to stem from sex-related biological differences [11]. Women can experience specific forms of depression, including; premenstrual dysphoric disorder (PMDD), postpartum and postmenopausal depression. These specific mental illnesses, in women, are associated with changes in ovarian hormones, and could contribute to the higher rate of psychiatric diseases in women [9].

The treatment of psychiatric illness during pregnancy and lactation is challenging, as most psychotropic drugs pose at least a hypothetical risk to the fetus and to the infant [15] while breastfeeding. The treatment of women with mental health problems during the perinatal period should be multidisciplinary and should include obstetricians and family practitioners.

4.2.1.2 Violence Against Women

In 1997, WHO declared Violence Against Women (VAW) a priority of health and a human rights concern. VAW was defined by the United Nations as [16]:

> *Any act of gender-based violence that results in, or is likely to result in, physical, sexual, or mental harm or suffering to women, including threats of such acts, coercion or arbitrary deprivation of liberty, whether occurring in public or in private life.* [16]

VAW is a serious public health problem globally, which is apparently under-reported in many countries. A multi-country study stated that 15–71% of women experienced VAW in their life. Most of these violent events are rarely disclosed [3].

VAW is an exceptionally complex phenomenon, being deep-rooted in many societies and cultures, with regards to a gender-based power of control, sexuality, identity and specific social customs and rules [17]. Negative outcomes of VAW, such as induced abortion, significantly affect both the physical and mental health of VAW victims [17].

The mental health consequences of VAW are extensive, with many victims suffering from damage to their own self-worth, following humiliation and entrapment. They lose a sense of self, the idea of a safe relationship, and of being loved and unharmed [18]. All those experiences involving such gender-based violence, result in increased rates of mental health problems. For example: depression, anxiety and post-traumatic stress disorder (PTSD) [18]. Almost all of their symptoms in women may persist longer than in men [18, 19], some victims of VAW attempt suicide after being exposed to trauma, especially sexual assault [20]. The rate of suicide in women is higher in countries, such as India, where virginity is considered an indicator of a woman's value [20].

With the recognition that VAW is a serious factor moderating health outcomes and a human rights issue, it is the duty of health providers to identify the problem, both mentally and physically, as to provide solutions to overcome these traumatic events [17]. Whilst, the root of VAW is deep and complex, social norms and cultural beliefs should be gradually changed by federal governments, to empower women both economically and socially [17]. Together, comprehensive health services and humanistic legal processes for victims should be provided to respond to these needs, empathically [3].

4.2.1.3 Gender Bias and Discrimination in Women

Many studies, regarding gender differences in medical treatment, reported gender bias in women's diagnosis and treatment, not limited to the psychiatric field. Generally female patients exhibit more symptoms than males, and these behaviors increase the physicians' tendency to prescribe, or switch drugs [21].

Cultural factors can have an effect on gender bias, regarding diagnosis and clinical management of psychiatric disorders. Individuals without a medical background may understand their symptoms differently compared to medical staff, coupled with this, physicians, including psychiatrists, may also misinterpret information. For instance; panic attacks in women are ordinarily viewed by local people, in southern Thailand, as usual "*women's problems*" called locally "*Wind Illness*" ("*Lom*"), and these symptoms according to local custom, do not require women to undergo any medical treatment [22]. On the other hand, if symptoms of a panic attack appear in men, both patients and doctors tend to react, and seek out medical support more appropriately [23].

The delay of treatment, based on gender bias, could also contribute to the higher rates of mental disease [1], especially in female adolescents, since, young people (10–25 years old) revealed more stigma, and under-diagnosis than adults, thus; innovative anti-stigma and mental- health, educational programs for youth may help reduce delay in the treatment of psychiatric disorders [24].

4.3 Gender Diversity and Mental Health

4.3.1 Other Gender Diversities, Specific Mental Illness and Risk Factors

The common phrase: "*lesbian, gay, bisexual, transgender and queer or questioning*" or LGBTQ, mentions a wide-ranging group of people, who are diverse in relation to their gender and sexual orientation [2]. LGBTQ, or other gender variants, are now accepted within what is generally considered to be the recognized spectrum of human experience [2]. So, health providers as well as other stakeholders should not focus on defining; "what type he/she is", but emphasize their gender identity and expression in addition to their individual perception, so as to provide proper health care [6].

Previous studies, in gender diversities and LGBTQ demonstrated, a significantly higher prevalence of mood, anxiety and substance-related disorders than that of the heterosexual population [6]. This mental distress is strongly related to suicidality, as LGBTQ individuals have been reported as having a higher rate of attempted suicides [25]. Adolescents, who have been identified as transgender are at the highest risk. [6]There is an acknowledged hypothesis that being LGBTQ is not fundamentally attributable to an increased risk of mental illness [7]. For example, well-being embedded as an internal conflict between an individual's appearance and identity, can lead to social stigma and rejection [7]. Severe social discrimination leads to a feeling of rejection and isolation, contributing to suicidality as a final conclusion [7].

Another factor contributing to mental illness, within the LGBTQ population, is problematic mental health services. Even in the US, mental health services for these specific populations are limited, and expert providers in the care of LGBTQ individuals are difficult to access [7]. Moreover, attitudes toward LGBTQ groups among mental health providers are not always genuinely positive. Hence, strong, non-judgmental collaboration between LGBTQ people and mental health providers could not always be established leading to worse outcomes [6].

4.3.2 *Gender Affirmation Care and Clinical Management*

The American academy of pediatrics (AAP) published a policy statement for the care of children, and adolescents with transgender identities along with other diverse genders [6]. Firstly, they are not categorized as psychiatric disorder patients, but a part of the recognized range of human variation [26]. The AAP also declared that the; "*reparative/conversion treatment*", which aims at changing young people's gender expression and identity, has been proven to be unsuccessful, unfair and inappropriate [27].

Secondly, any mental problem that exists among LGBTQ youths, always stems from negative experiences and social stigma, not their own intrinsic being [6]. Thus, the AAP suggested the gender-affirmation care model (GACM), to offer proper care for children and adolescents, by integrating health providers and social services [5]. The primary goal is to destigmatize gender diversity, and appreciate their gender experience in order to encourage their self- worth [5]. Therefore, the therapists of GACM have a duty to assist them to encourage skills for dealing with gender-based discrimination, and stigma [5]. Regarding the GACM model, pediatric and mental health providers have an important role to educate families, and promote safe communities where any child can develop and explore their own gender, liberally [5]. Finally, every intervention of GACM must focus on LGBTQ youth's physical and cognitive development, individually [6].

Many guidelines and protocols recommended that gender development should be a part of routine wellness child visits. Since, pediatric primary care providers are often the first ones who recognize gender identity, and gender-related distress in children [6]. However, the recommended way to approach LGBTQ individuals, in every age group, is direct inquiry and non-judgmental questions about their gender-related experiences as well as feelings [28].

To avoid exacerbating gender dysphoria, and so as to not contribute to more stigmatization; pediatricians, medical and mental health providers should be aware of their own expertise and attitudes towards LGBTQ people. If any provider does not feel comfortable for caring for these specific populations, referral to another provider with more expertise is applicable [6].

4.3.3 Gender Bias and Discrimination

Social status of LGBTQ groups has been considered the "other" in society, because they cannot fit in normative gender roles, or perceived according to cultural expectations [2]. Being: "*otherness*", by traditional worldviews is the root of stigmatization, bias and discrimination, much the same as psychiatric patients [29]. Due to social stigma, they are fearful of the provider's discrimination, and have concerns on safety issues; hence, 1 in 4 LGBTQ adults avoid compulsory visits to health care services, and LGBTQ individuals are now facing health disparities and obstacles within the health care system. [30] The inequity in health care services, regarding gender-based identity and expression, is viewed with apprehension by world-wide professional medical organizations, and federal governments [8].

However, to be more humanistic and holistic; "*a life-course perspective*", is the recommended framework for health providers to identify individual LGBTQ needs, and to appreciate their experiences, which are determined by their historical and socio-economical context. (e.g. family, peers, neighborhoods and colleagues) [4]. The clinical skills for approaching along with understanding gender diversity requires knowledge-based experience. Thus, medical-associated curriculums, multi-disciplinary and residency training programs should emphasize gender identity related issues in the fields of pediatrics, psychiatry, family medicine, obstetrics and gynecology [31].

The AAP also pointed out that it is the role of all health care providers, educators and school administrators to educate communities, and promote acceptance of gender diversity [6]. A survey in 2015 showed that specific anti-bullying policies and curriculums in school including positive representations of LGBTQ groups, resulted in less hostility toward LGBTQ youths at school [32]. Hence, school staff also have an essential duty to recognize and prevent bullying at school. More than half of LGBTQ students were reported as having suffered gender-based harassment, and they stated that greater connections to school staff created a better sense of security [32].

4.3.4 Remarks

Gender inequality has been disparaging globally both towards the physical and mental health of women, and other genders for centuries [20]. Many socio-cultural contexts provide men with more resources, influence and authority [17]. Improvement of gender equity in mental health is one of the straightest, and most effective ways to reduce mental health inequities. Constant, effective human rights implementation, and powerful reinforcement should be used as an influential mechanism to motivate both governments and people [3, 8]. Most of all, women, along with other genders themselves, must be encouraged to take more control and to recognize their own rights, including mental health service access [3, 8].

To inspire and educate people, the elementary values and beliefs of gender equality, especially regarding mental health, should begin from fundamental, educational systems [6]. School, educators and administrators must emphasize gender-based harassment, and discrimination as an unacceptable issue [31]. Moreover, educational curriculums should teach students about gender diversity, wherein; not only gender-binary or "*only men and women*" exist on earth [2]. On the other hand, gender diversity (or the LGBTQ population) are a part of the normal spectrum of human condition [26]. Gradually, positive representations of LGBTQ people, included in higher curriculums could de-stigmatise and increase feelings of safety among LGBTQ students at school [31]. Along with helping them find a sense of acceptance and belonging through meaningful connections with peers [30]. Anti-bullying policies should be promoted in order to protect, not only female and other genders, but also other valuable populations.

Primary health care services have an important role in enhancing their competencies to recognize the mental health consequences of violence against women (VAW) as well as other genders [3]. When VAW, or gender-based harassment occurs, the key framework is multidisciplinary collaboration among families, health care providers, law-enforcement, and social services [17]. Psychological support from these teams is an essential, protective factor to prevent mental illness in these populations [3]. Long-term follow-up of mental health problems is recommended, since VAW tends to produce long-lasting psychiatric symptoms, such as PTSD. Hence, social provision, health care services and judicial processes should try their best to avoid re-traumatizing victims by the system. However, more research on '*resilience*' following such violence and harassment against women, trans-gender and other diversities is currently needed for developing evidence-based recovery programs. [33]

As the American academy of pediatrics recommended; child psychiatrists and pediatricians should understand their role regarding gender diversities, and improve expertise of the developmental aspects of gender identity, gender perception, gender expression and sexual orientation of both children and adolescents [6]. To categorize LGBTQ youths, using derogatory terminology; like, the term "*Cherry*" used in Thailand to identify a female identity but whom are sexually attracted to homosexual males, is unacceptable in any healthcare environment [34]. It is an outdated and a deceptive approach that would produce more social stigma from health care providers [29, 30]. Evidence-based research is currently required to influence policy makers for providing statements of expenditure about women and other genders in mental health care, and providing laws against gender-based discrimination and violence.

4.4   Brief Conclusion

Women and gender diversity in mental health care are currently a concern for many professional health organizations, because gender is an important factor for several dimensions of mental difficulties. Even though some women's psychiatric problems stem from biological differences, such as; hormonal changes, some psycho-social aspects; for example, violence against women, also have a strong effect on various mental disorders. Mental difficulties among people with diverse gender identities (or LGBTQ) mostly arise from negative experiences and traumatic discrimination. Although, gender diversity is currently considered within the recognized spectrum of human condition.

Therefore, gender equality is the key solution to promote mental health among these populations. Gender-based bias and harassment are utterly unacceptable, along with mental health disparities. However, mental health providers need multi-disciplinary collaborations coupled with knowledge-based experience for the care of women, and LGBTQ individuals. It is applicable to refer to another expert, when a provider feels unprepared to approach and care for these populations. There are many gaps in knowledge about mental health in women and gender diverse populations, hence; research is still required.

Future Tasks

- Understanding of gender diversity and sexual orientation must be promoted for acceptance without fear of harassment or bullying, as a part of basic national education
- The curriculum of mental health and psychiatry, for undergraduate study and postgraduate training for all health professionals, should consider integrating competencies of practices for caring of women, trans-gender peoples and other gender diversities.
- Multidisciplinary and collaborative approaches for the clinical assessment of gender identity and violence against women, should be implemented in all medical settings. However, in low resource countries this approach must be adapted appropriately
- Primary care providers, mental health workers, educators, school administrators and mass media in each country should meet together for discussions on their important roles in promoting policies, and laws to prevent gender-based discrimination along with violence against women
- Upcoming studies and research are needed for evidence-based care of women, and other genders to influence policies of gender equality as well as laws against discrimination and violence, regarding both gender identity and expression.

References

1. World Health Organization. (2018). *Gender and women's mental health*. World Health Organization. http://www.who.int/mental_health/prevention/genderwomen/en/. Accessed 2 Nov 2018.
2. Institute of Medicine (US) Committee on Lesbian, Gay, Bisexual, and Transgender Health Issues and Research Gaps and Opportunities. (2018). *The health of lesbian, gay, bisexual, and transgender people: Building a foundation for better understanding*. National Academies Press (US). https://www.ncbi.nlm.nih.gov/books/NBK64806. Accessed 2 Nov 2018.
3. World Health Organization. *Violence against women*. World Health Organization 2017. http://www.who.int/en/news-room/fact-sheets/detail/violence-against-women. Accessed 10 Nov 2018.
4. Cohler, B., & Hammack, P. (2007). The psychological world of the gay teenager: Social change, narrative, and "Normality". *Journal of Youth and Adolescence, 36*, 47–59.
5. Glynn, T. R., Gamarel, K. E., Kahler, C. W., Iwamoto, M., Operario, D., & Nemoto, T. (2016). The role of gender affirmation in psychological well-being among transgender women. *Psychology of Sexual Orientation and Gender Diversity, 3*, 336–344.
6. Rafferty, J. (2018). Ensuring comprehensive care and support for transgender and gender-diverse children and adolescents. *Pediatrics*. http://pediatrics.aappublications.org/content/142/4/e20182162. Accessed 20 Oct 2018.
7. Edwards-Leeper, L., & Spack, N. P. (2012). Psychological evaluation and medical treatment of transgender youth in an interdisciplinary "Gender Management Service" (GeMS) in a major pediatric center. *Journal of Homosexuality, 59*, 321–336.
8. World Health Organization. *Women and gender equity*. World Health Organization 2018. https://www.who.int/social_determinants/themes/womenandgender/en/66. Accessed 10 Nov 2018.
9. Gordon, J. L., & Girdler, S. S. (2014). Hormone replacement therapy in the treatment of peri-menopausal depression. *Current Psychiatry Reports, 16*, 517–527.
10. National Health Service Digital. (2018). *Adult psychiatric morbidity survey: Survey of mental health and wellbeing, England, 2014*. NHS Digital. https://digital.nhs.uk/data-and-information/publications/statistical/adult-psychiatric-morbidity-survey/adult-psychiatric-morbidity-survey-survey-of-mental-health-and-wellbeing-england-2014. Accessed 14 Nov 2018.
11. Albert, P. (2015). Why is depression more prevalent in women? *Journal of Psychiatry & Neuroscience, 40*, 219–221.
12. Patten, S. B., Wang, J. L., Williams, J. V., Currie, S., Beck, C. A., Maxwell, C. J., et al. (2006). Descriptive epidemiology of major depression in Canada. *Canadian Journal of Psychiatry, 51*, 84–90.
13. Arnold, L. M. (2003). Gender differences in bipolar disorder. *The Psychiatric Clinics of North America, 26*, 595–620.
14. McGrath, J., Saha, S., Welham, J., El Saadi, O., MacCauley, C., & Chant, D. (2004). A systematic review of the incidence of schizophrenia: The distribution of rates and the influence of sex, urbanicity, migrant status and methodology. *BMC Medicine, 2*, 13. https://bmcmedicine.biomedcentral.com/articles/10.1186/1741-7015-2-13 Accessed 14 Nov 2018.
15. Parial, S. (2015). Bipolar disorder in women. *Indian Journal of Psychiatry, 57*, 252–263.
16. World Health Organization. *Global and regional estimates of violence against women*. World Health Organization 2013. https://www.who.int/reproductivehealth/publications/violence/9789241564625/en/. Accessed 17 Nov 2018.
17. Kumar, A., Haque Nizamie, S., & Srivastava, N. K. (2013). Violence against women and mental health. *Mental Health & Prevention, 1*, 4–10.
18. Brown, G. W., Harris TO, & Hepworth, C. (1995). Loss, humiliation and entrapment among women developing depression: A patient and non-patient comparison. *Psychological Medicine, 25*, 7–21.
19. Jatchavala, C., & Vittayanont, A. (2017). Post-traumatic stress disorder symptoms among patients with substance-related disorders in the restive areas of south Thailand insurgency. *Songklanagarind Medical Journal, 35*, 121–132.

20. Kumar, S., Jeyaseelan, L., Suresh, S., & Ahuja, R. C. (2005). Domestic violence and its mental health correlates in Indian women. *The British Journal of Psychiatry, 187*, 62–67.
21. Safran, D. G., Rogers, W. H., Tarlov, A. R., McHorney, C. A., & Ware, J. (1997). Gender differences in medical treatment: The case of physician-prescribed activity restrictions. *Social Science & Medicine, 45*, 711–722.
22. Udomratn, P., & Hinton, D. (2009). Gendered panic in southern Thailand: '*lom*' ("wind") illness and '*wuup*' ("upsurge") illness. In D. Hinton & B. Good (Eds.), *Culture and panic disorder* (pp. 183–204). California: Stanford University Press.
23. Udomratn, P. (2000). Panic disorder in Thailand: A report on the secondary data analysis. *Journal of the Medical Association of Thailand, 83*, 1158–1166.
24. Kutcher, S., Bagnell, A., & Wei, Y. (2015). Mental health literacy in secondary schools: A Canadian approach. *Child and Adolescent Psychiatric Clinics of North America, 24*, 233–244.
25. Sutter, M., & Perrin, P. B. (2016). Discrimination, mental health, and suicidal ideation among LGBTQ people of color. *Journal of Counseling Psychology, 63*, 98–105.
26. Bonifacio, H. J., & Rosenthal, S. M. (2015). Gender variance and dysphoria in children and adolescents. *Pediatric Clinics of North America, 62*, 1001–1016.
27. American Academy of Pediatrics, California. (2018). *Sexual orientation: Change efforts [Internet]*. California: Aap-ca.org. http://aap-ca.org/bill/sexual-orientation-change-efforts-2/. Accessed 20 Nov 2018.
28. Ehrensaft, D. (2017). Gender nonconforming youth: Current perspectives. *Adolescent Health, Medicine and Therapeutics, 8*, 57–67.
29. Jatchavala, C. (2013). Discourse and stigmatization of psychiatric disorder in Thailand. *Journal of Sociology and Anthropology, 33*, 94–113.
30. Fedchuk, D. (2017). *Majorities within minorities: The experiences of non-suicidal self-injury in the LGBTQ communities* [Master of Science]. Massey University of New Zealand.
31. Obedin-Maliver, J., Goldsmith, E., Stewart, L., White, W., Tran, E., Brenman, S., et al. (2011). Lesbian, gay, bisexual, and transgender-related content in undergraduate medical education. *JAMA, 306*, 971–977.
32. Kosciw, D. (2018). *The 2015 National School Climate Survey: The experiences of lesbian, gay, bisexual, transgender, and queer youth in our nation's schools*. Executive summary. https://eric.ed.gov/?id=ED574808. Accessed 21 Nov 2018.
33. Kwon, P. (2013). Resilience in lesbian, gay, and bisexual individuals. *Personality and Social Psychology Review, 17*(4), 371–383.
34. General, R. (2018). *Thailand has 18 different gender identities*. NextShark. http://nextshark.com/thailand-18-different-gender-identities/. Accessed 24 Nov 2018.

Chapter 5
Diversity and Gender Differences in Treatment

Blanca Bolea-Alamanac

Key Points
- Sex bias and sex omission are still present in mental health research in general and pharmacological research in particular, despite some progress in the last decade.
- Minorities face several barriers to access healthcare and are often under-represented in clinical trials.
- Psychological treatments are not devoid of gender biases and require specific adjustments to engage men.
- Cultural adaptations of psychotherapeutic interventions increase acceptability and engagement by ethnic minorities and can be more effective than their non-adapted counterparts.
- Equity in treatment produces positive effects that cascade to society at large.
- Special attention to women's mental health in the perinatal period is required, effective treatment in this key phase of the lives of women and children has long-lasting positive effects.
- To achieve mental health interventions that reach all communities and encompass both genders, engagement at all levels is necessary, including consultation with stakeholders, inclusion of minorities in the research discourse, directives by funding and regulatory institutions and diverse, gender balanced research teams.

B. Bolea-Alamanac (✉)
University of Toronto, Women's College Hospital and Centre for Addiction and Mental Health, WCH Institute for Health System Solutions and Virtual Care (WIHV), Toronto, ON, Canada

© The Author(s) 2019
S. Bährer-Kohler, B. Bolea-Alamanac (eds.), *Diversity in Global Mental Health*, SpringerBriefs in Psychology, https://doi.org/10.1007/978-3-030-29112-9_5

5.1   Introduction

Despite some progress in recent years, the general assumption of the male gender
as normative and the female gender as the exception is widespread. In research,
studies with limited funding that involve complex procedures tend to recruit a male
population first and only later if relevant effects are found are these studies repli-
cated in women [1]. This has limited greatly our understanding of neurological
pathways in the brain that may differ by sex. For the purpose of this chapter sex bias
will be defined as the favoring of one sex against the other while sex omission will
be defined as the lack of reporting by sex [2]. Same challenges apply to the inclusion of minorities in research. The lack of representation of all the populations
where research is undertaken inevitably leads to treatments that are biased towards
one sex and/or one specific ethnicity. This fact not only compromises the applicabil-
ity of treatments and medical procedures to the general population, but it also affects
what topics or areas are considered worthy of study from a funding perspective.
Most medical research is biased towards problems faced in the Northern/Western
hemisphere and by a population of predominantly middle-class citizens that can
afford some type of health coverage or live in countries where the government
provides health services [3]. In this chapter the various challenges regarding the
treatment of a diverse and gender balanced population will be reviewed with a special emphasis on what strategies can help to develop inclusive treatments and
interventions.

5.2   Content

5.2.1   Sex Bias in Pharmacological Research

A cardinal pitfall of pharmacological research is the lack of equal recruitment of
both sexes in experimental studies. Preclinical studies suffer from lack of sex balanced designs [2, 4]. Most animal studies include male animal models only and
when this is not the case, results are not always reported by sex [4]. This bias has
also been found in research involving human cell lines [5]. The absence of basic
research on female models of disease limits the generalization of these results to
both sexes in subsequent phases of research. If a compound is only tried in a male
animal and is not found useful it is unlikely to progress to tests in female models. It
is often considered that because it is not useful in one sex is unlikely to be valuable
in the other. The same can be assumed for side effects. Compounds that are only
tested in one sex cannot be safely used in both [6].

   The standard procedure to prove effectiveness of a drug in humans after
research in animals is a Randomized Control Trial (RCT). A randomized controlled trial is a type of experimental paradigm where two groups of individuals
that are comparable in terms of illness receive either a placebo (a medication

without an active compound) or the targeted medication and then are evaluated blindly (neither the subject nor the clinicians know what the patient has taken), in order to ascertain if the medication has a positive effect. Regulatory bodies will examine the results of RCTs before a medication is granted a license for a specific indication. It is a well-known fact that human trials in pharmacology often fail to recruit equal numbers of women and men [7]. Several funding and regulatory bodies have tackled this problem by enforcing policies that mandate the inclusion of women [8]. Despite progress towards equal recruitment, reporting on the results of drug RCTs by gender has been slow [9, 10]. A review of one hundred and seven studies published in fourteen high impact medical journals found that the mean of female enrollment was 47% (considering only studies of non-sex specific ill-nesses). This is an increase in recruitment of almost 10 points from previous data obtained a decade ago [9], even though 15% of the studies sampled enrolled less than 30% of women [10]. Sex omission persists, 77% of the studies sampled did not include sex as a covariate in the analysis nor reported results by sex. The unequal representation and reporting of results by sex in clinical trials may explain the higher rates of side effects or lack of response to treatment in women versus men seen in post-marketing data of some drugs [6, 10, 11], highlighting the risks of sex bias in research. Differences by sex have been found in the absorption, distribution, metabolism and elimination of drugs [12]. When data is obtained from both sexes and analyzed accordingly, these disparities become evident [6]. A classic example is the case of a hypnotic drug used for insomnia, which can stay in the blood stream of women twice as long as in men, producing at the same dose a stronger sedative effect and requiring different dosing in men and women [13]. Another medication, an opioid antagonist used to reduce the risk of relapse in patients treated for alcohol misuse [14] may have opposite effects in women and men with comorbid drug abuse increasing use of cocaine and alcohol in women and decreasing use of both substances in men [14]. Sex differences have also been detected in other types of treatments such as electroconvulsive therapy (ECT) which is an efficient and rapid treatment for certain severe psychiatric conditions such as major depression when pharmacological and psychological treatments have failed. Some studies have showed that women require less dose (charge intensity in this case) and both sexes require higher doses according to age [15].

5.3   Research on Psychiatric Treatments and Diverse Populations

Minorities are underrepresented in clinical research [16]. A review of more than 300 clinical trials for depression in the US found that despite recent improvements in inclusion, minority ethnic groups were still underrepresented [17]. Another study found that only 13% of published RCTs in high impact journals described results by ethnicity and when it was reported patients of Afro-American descent and Hispanic subjects were underrepresented [9, 10]. Linguistic minorities and recent immigrants are also frequently overlooked [17]. The lack of recruitment of minorities means that effects that can be moderated by factors related specifically to those communities such as differences in diet, social or culturally related habits or genetic differences cannot be evaluated [18]. For example, the metabolic activity of some liver enzymes (the chemical compounds that break down drugs in the liver) vary by ethnicity [19, 20] and not including a diverse population in drug trials may underestimate these effects [21, 22]. Studies also show that minorities have less access to certain complex therapies such as electroconvulsive therapy (ECT) [23] accessibility problems adding to the lack of evidence. Previous unethical research conducted in ethnic minorities [24] has created an atmosphere of distrust between researchers and communities that requires reflective and careful bridging. Another relevant issue is the fact that in recent years, pharmaceutical companies have progressively moved operations to developing countries where recruitment of patients may be easier because of lower access to care which in itself raises major ethical, legal and humanitarian questions [25].

5.4 Psychological Treatments, Sex Bias and Diversity

Psychological treatments are not devoid of sex and ethnicity biases. Psychological interventions are influenced by the socio-cultural constructs of those that develop them, as well as those of the clients they target. Most psychotherapies use cultural paradigms that may not be applicable outside the sphere of Western Anglo-Saxon culture [3]. The appearance of mindfulness-based interventions, a type of therapy that is rooted in Buddhish practices [26] being one of the few transcultural elements that have been assimilated to mainstream treatment in recent years. There has been a paucity of research on differential effects of psychological treatments across ethnicities [27]. Some authors have highlighted the need to include cultural elements in the adaptation of psychological programs to specific communities [28]. This culturally adapted interventions can have trickle down effects, engaging marginalized communities, enhancing communication between health care providers and users and decreasing stigma by creating a conversation in the community about mental health [29]. Delivering interventions by including them in an activity that is socially acceptable for that community is a creative and efficient way of promoting health [30]. Examples of this integration include using dance as part of a rehabilitative intervention in older adults of Hispanic descent [31] and the use of sweat lodges as part of integrative care in First Nation's patients [32].

Regarding gender differences in psychotherapy, and in contrast with preclinical and pharmacological research, most studies show greater effects of psychological treatment in women [33, 34] than men. This is probably mediated by social gender roles and less treatment seeking and engagement in psychosocial treatments by men outside court mandated interventions [35]. Several barriers are evident such as social pressure forcing men to not communicate their mental state, difficulty taking time off work for treatment when they are the main breadwinner and stigma [33]. Interventions to increase men's engagement in therapy include adding gender sensitive techniques that explore the patient's view of his masculinity, use of appropriate nonjudgmental metaphors and establishing goals that respect the patient's gender perceptions [36]. In the last decade a larger conversation has appeared highlighting the importance of teaching children of both genders about emotional communication and emotional regulation [37]. This is likely to reduce stigma around seeking help in men as well as increase communication about wellness and mental health in general.

5.5 The Benefits of Gender Equity in Treatment

Society at large benefits from addressing women's mental health needs. Women are the main caregiver in most of the world. If women do not have access to mental health care, children and other dependents suffer too. The most obvious effects are probably seen in perinatal interventions. Several studies have found an association between depression and anxiety during pregnancy and the post-natal period and children's mental health [38]. Post-natal depression for example is linked to higher infant mortality, morbidity and risk of neglect [39]. Several interventions have been used to increase the identification and treatment of women in the perinatal period, including educational campaigns for the public and medical staff, routine screening by obstetric teams of depression symptoms using validated measures and social interventions where specific support is provided by health care professionals during the perinatal period. One study found that daughters of women who had access to a specialized nurse visiting them at home up to 4 years after delivery had significantly less risk of being involved in the justice system at age 19 than those whose mothers were not offered the extra support [40]. Proving that the effects of increasing access to health care in women and particularly mental health care can produce waterfall effects for the community. Another relevant benefit is that women are effective communicators and can act as a network of support and source of education for the family and the community at large. Interventions that give women a voice and empower them have proved effectiveness at societal level [41].

5.6 Discussion: Towards Gender Inclusive and Intersectional Treatments

Several strategies can be put in place to obtain appropriate representation of women and minorities in clinical trials and research in general. Guidelines and policies that address gender and diversity should be developed and enforced at various levels, from regulatory organizations and funding bodies to clinical journals. A recent study found that scientific journals that had policies as regards to reporting results by sex had more articles where this variable was included in the analysis and results [10]. A review of sex bias in neuroscience research recommended considering the explicit inclusion of both sexes as a positive factor to obtain funding [4]. Demythologizing false beliefs that have impaired research in female animal models is important as well as not limiting that research to reproductive oriented only experiments. Battling the cognitive bias that sets the female as the exception and the white Caucasian man as the norm is particularly relevant. Women outnumber men after the age of 55 worldwide [42], however treatments for illnesses that increase with age are still typically tested in predominantly male samples. Issues around pregnancy and fertility are unlikely to be a barrier in this specific population proving that gender biases are at play. Informing and educating researchers, decision makers and funding organizations is vital. Ethics committees should be aware that studies that exclude women without a clear rationale and inherently unethical [43]. Funding bodies should encourage recruitment of both sexes and provide incentives to researchers to change practices [4].

A multidisciplinary approach is required to increase recruitment of minorities in clinical trials [44] which should include addressing common barriers reported by these populations to both access health care in general and clinical trials in particular. These barriers include lack of insurance, absence of information in the patient's main language, lack of representation from the community targeted in the development of research projects and difficulties related to socioeconomic status [44]. In recent years, researchers have included user representation in the development of protocols and this has led to a positive sense of ownership of research projects by communities than otherwise would be marginalized [45]. Knowing what problems these communities identify as regards to mental health and what their priorities are in terms of treatment is a first step [46]. In the case of psychotherapy, culturally adapted interventions have proved more effective in ethnic minorities [47]. Cultural adaptation is defined as a modification of a psychological paradigm to include beliefs, practices and social constructs relevant to a particular community. These should include but are not limited to, language changes or culturally equivalent translations, acknowledgement of those values relevant for the specific population and cultural safety practices. For example, a culturally adapted parent training intervention for Hispanic patients that acknowledged the migratory experience and bilingualism of these patients showed high levels of acceptability [48] while a culturally adapted intervention for Asian Americans with phobias was proved superior to a non-adapted manualized therapy [49]. Outreach of academic results to the community and specifically to minorities will help them access care and participate in further studies creating long-lasting relationships between researchers and stakeholders [50]. Community rooted initiatives to develop and communicate results of research such as CBKT (Community Based Knowledge Translation) recognize that civil societies (from advocacy groups to neighborhood associations) have a role in healthcare and research. Community partnerships are at the core of such efforts.

A case study of this approach is the Social Networking App- Action for Resilience (SONAR) initiative. This project aimed to improve social interconnectedness in a small rural Canadian town. Community stakeholders (including the town and First Nations council) and local youth were included in the decision process from the project's beginning. Community leaders, youth representatives and researchers brainstormed together and this work led to the development of a smart phone app that would synthesize available mental health and healthy local leisure resources, allow users to post and share ideas to improve their community and provide information about evidence based interventions for mental health problems [51].

Diversity and the intersectionality of this diversity should not be reduced to the individuals participating in research studies. Women are still exposed to significant societal, institutional and family related challenges that impair their professional progress in the field of science [52], despite graduating in many disciplines in higher numbers than men. Women are still excluded from positions of power [53]. There is also a lack of visibility for female scientists [54], which leads to a lack of role models to inspire younger generations and lack of recognition. Inclusion of women and ethnic minorities in research teams and in the organizational structure and hierarchy of research institutions is necessary in order to have a wider vision on what health/mental health gaps should be targeted by research and what the priorities should be for an inclusive and equal society.

5.7 Conclusion

In this chapter the main challenges for the development of psychiatric treatments from a gender and diversity point of view have been summarized. Preclinical research is still based on male models of illness. Minorities are underrepresented in clinical trials. Sex omission in the reporting of research results is common, even if recruitment of women in research has improved. These leads to an increase rate of side effects and lack of efficacy of treatments in women and minorities. Research that acknowledges the importance of sex balanced samples, reports and analyzes results by gender and that is inclusive is required. This is particularly relevant because effective treatment of mental health problems in women cascades to the community creating positive intergenerational effects. Researchers can be incentivized to act on these issues by several means including professional guidelines, directives issued by funding bodies and stricter editorial processes. Community involvement and partnerships with stakeholders are key in the development of inclusive interventions. Gender balanced, and culturally and ethnically diverse staff is also necessary. Gold standard treatments in mental health consider the individual in its ecological context and should provide medication, psychological therapy and social support that are tailored to the patient's needs and the needs of the communities they serve.

Future Tasks

- Funding bodies, research institutions, editorial boards and researchers at large should be aware of the existence of sex bias and sex omission in research and promote research practices that are inclusive of both genders.
- Treatments that are gender and ethnicity-aware are likely to be more effective.
- Addressing mental health difficulties in women during the perinatal period can have positive 'cascading' intergenerational effects.
- Partnerships and collaborations with stakeholders in the community as well as investigating the reasons why minorities do not engage in research is vital to bridge the gap in healthcare that affects this population.

Bibliography

1. Lind, K. E., Gutierrez, E. J., Yamamoto, D. J., Regner, M. F., McKee, S. A., & Tanabe, J. (2017). Sex disparities in substance abuse research: Evaluating 23 years of structural neuroimaging studies. *Drug and Alcohol Dependence, 173*, 92–98.
2. Will, T. R., Proano, S. B., Thomas, A. M., Kunz, L. M., Thompson, K. C., Ginnari, L. A., Jones, C. H., Lucas, S. C., Reavis, E. M., Dorris, D. M., & Meitzen, J. (2017). Problems and progress regarding sex bias and omission in neuroscience research. *eNeuro, 4*(6), ENEURO.0278–ENEU17.2017.
3. Nielsen, M., Haun, D., Kartner, J., & Legare, C. H. (2017). The persistent sampling bias in developmental psychology: A call to action. *Journal of Experimental Child Psychology, 162*, 31–38.
4. Beery, A. K., & Zucker, I. (2011). Sex bias in neuroscience and biomedical research. *Neuroscience and Biobehavioral Reviews, 35*(3), 565–572.
5. Kong, B. Y., Haugh, I. M., Schlosser, B. J., Getsios, S., & Paller, A. S. (2016). Mind the gap: Sex bias in basic skin research. *The Journal of Investigative Dermatology, 136*(1), 12–14.
6. GAO. (2001). *Most drugs withdrawn in recent years had greater health risks for women.* https://www.gao.gov/products/GAO-01-286R. Accessed 16 Dec 2018.
7. Phillips, S. P., & Hamberg, K. (2016). Doubly blind: A systematic review of gender in randomised controlled trials. *Global Health Action, 9*, 29597. https://doi.org/10.3402/gha.v3409.29597.
8. FDA. (1993). Guideline for the study and evaluation of gender differences in the clinical evaluation of drugs; notice. *Federal Register, 58*(139), 39406–39416.
9. Geller, S. E., Koch, A., Pellettieri, B., & Carnes, M. (2011). Inclusion, analysis, and reporting of sex and race/ethnicity in clinical trials: Have we made progress? *Journal of Women's Health (2002), 20*(3), 315–320.
10. Geller, S. E., Koch, A. R., Roesch, P., Filut, A., Hallgren, E., & Carnes, M. (2018). The more things change, the more they stay the same: A study to evaluate compliance with inclusion and assessment of women and minorities in randomized controlled trials. *Academic Medicine : Journal of the Association of American Medical Colleges, 93*(4), 630–635.
11. Fisher, J. A., & Ronald, L. M. (2010). Sex, gender, and pharmaceutical politics: From drug development to marketing. *Gender Medicine, 7*(4), 357–370.

12. Marazziti, D., Baroni, S., Picchetti, M., Piccinni, A., Carlini, M., Vatteroni, E., Falaschi, V., Lombardi, A., & Dell'Osso, L. (2013). Pharmacokinetics and pharmacodinamics of psychotropic drugs: Effect of sex. *CNS Spectrums, 18*(3), 118–127.
13. Verster, J. C., & Roth, T. (2012). Gender differences in highway driving performance after administration of sleep medication: A review of the literature. *Traffic Injury Prevention, 13*(3), 286–292.
14. Pettinati, H. M., Kampman, K. M., Lynch, K. G., Suh, J. J., Dackis, C. A., Oslin, D. W., & O'Brien, C. P. (2008). Gender differences with high-dose naltrexone in patients with co-occurring cocaine and alcohol dependence. *Journal of Substance Abuse Treatment, 34*(4), 378–390.
15. Salvador Sanchez, J., David, M. D., Torrent Seto, A., Martinez Alonso, M., Portella Moll, M. J., Pifarre Paredero, J., Vieta Pascual, E., & Mur Lain, M. (2017). Electroconvulsive therapy clinical database: Influence of age and gender on the electrical charge. *Revista de psiquiatria y salud mental, 10*(3), 143–148.
16. Chen, M. S., Jr., Lara, P. N., Dang, J. H., Paterniti, D. A., & Kelly, K. (2014). Twenty years post-NIH Revitalization Act: Enhancing minority participation in clinical trials (EMPaCT): Laying the groundwork for improving minority clinical trial accrual: Renewing the case for enhancing minority participation in cancer clinical trials. *Cancer, 120 Suppl 7*, 1091–1096.
17. Polo, A. J., Makol, B. A., Castro, A. S., Colon-Quintana, N., Wagstaff, A. E., & Guo, S. (2019). Diversity in randomized clinical trials of depression: A 36-year review. *Clinical Psychology Review, 67*, 22–35.
18. A, L. L., Naranjo, M. E., Rodrigues-Soares, F., Penas, L. E. M., Farinas, H., & Tarazona-Santos, E. (2014). Interethnic variability of CYP2D6 alleles and of predicted and measured metabolic phenotypes across world populations. *Expert Opinion on Drug Metabolism & Toxicology, 10*(11), 1569–1583.
19. Cespedes-Garro, C., Fricke-Galindo, I., Naranjo, M. E., Rodrigues-Soares, F., Farinas, H., de Andres, F., Lopez-Lopez, M., Penas-Lledo, E. M., & LL, A. (2015). Worldwide interethnic variability and geographical distribution of CYP2C9 genotypes and phenotypes. *Expert Opinion on Drug Metabolism & Toxicology, 11*(12), 1893–1905.
20. Gaedigk, A., Sangkuhl, K., Whirl-Carrillo, M., Klein, T., & Leeder, J. S. (2016). Prediction of CYP2D6 phenotype from genotype across world populations. *Genetics in Medicine, 19*, 69.
21. Denisenko, N. P., Sychev, D. A., Sizova, Z. M., Rozhkov, A. V., & Kondrashov, A. V. (2016). Effect of CYP2C19 genetic polymorphisms on the efficacy of proton pump inhibitor-based triple eradication therapy in Slavic patients with peptic ulcers: A meta-analysis. *Eksperimental'naia i klinicheskaia gastroenterologiia (Experimental & Clinical Gastroenterology)*, (11), 11–16.
22. Giri, A. K., Khan, N. M., Grover, S., Kaur, I., Basu, A., Tandon, N., Scaria, V., Kukreti, R., Brahmachari, S. K., & Bharadwaj, D. (2014). Genetic epidemiology of pharmacogenetic variations in CYP2C9, CYP4F2 and VKORC1 genes associated with warfarin dosage in the Indian population. *Pharmacogenomics, 15*(10), 1337–1354.
23. Breakey, W. R., & Dunn, G. J. (2004). Racial disparity in the use of ECT for affective disorders. *The American Journal of Psychiatry, 161*(9), 1635–1641.
24. Weindling, P., von Villiez, A., Loewenau, A., & Farron, N. (2016). The victims of unethical human experiments and coerced research under National Socialism. *Endeavour, 40*(1), 1–6.
25. Weigmann, K. (2015). The ethics of global clinical trials: In developing countries, participation in clinical trials is sometimes the only way to access medical treatment. What should be done to avoid exploitation of disadvantaged populations? *EMBO Reports, 16*(5), 566–570.
26. Sipe, W. E., & Eisendrath, S. J. (2012). Mindfulness-based cognitive therapy: Theory and practice. *Canadian Journal of Psychiatry (Revue canadienne de psychiatrie), 57*(2), 63–69.
27. Tao, K. W., Owen, J., Pace, B. T., & Imel, Z. E. (2015). A meta-analysis of multicultural competencies and psychotherapy process and outcome. *Journal of Counseling Psychology, 62*(3), 337–350.

28. Mehl-Madrona, L. (2016). Indigenous knowledge approach to successful psychotherapies with aboriginal suicide attempters. *Canadian Journal of Psychiatry (Revue canadienne de psychiatrie), 61*(11), 696–699.
29. Calabria, B., Clifford, A., Rose, M., & Shakeshaft, A. P. (2014). Tailoring a family-based alcohol intervention for Aboriginal Australians, and the experiences and perceptions of health care providers trained in its delivery. *BMC Public Health, 14*, 322.
30. Eley, R., & Gorman, D. (2010). Didgeridoo playing and singing to support asthma management in Aboriginal Australians. *The Journal of Rural Health, 26*(1), 100–104.
31. Marquez, D. X., Wilson, R., Aguinaga, S., Vasquez, P., Fogg, L., Yang, Z., Wilbur, J., Hughes, S., & Spanbauer, C. (2017). Regular Latin dancing and health education may improve cognition of late middle-aged and older Latinos. *Journal of Aging and Physical Activity, 25*(3), 482–489.
32. Schiff, J. W., & Moore, K. (2006). The impact of the sweat lodge ceremony on dimensions of well-being. *American Indian and Alaska Native Mental Health Research (Online), 13*(3), 48–69.
33. Krysinska, K., Batterham, P. J., & Christensen, H. (2017). Differences in the effectiveness of psychosocial interventions for suicidal ideation and behaviour in women and men: A systematic review of randomised controlled trials. *Archives of Suicide Research, 21*(1), 12–32.
34. Kvarstein, E. H., Nordviste, O., Dragland, L., & Wilberg, T. (2017). Outpatient psychodynamic group psychotherapy - outcomes related to personality disorder, severity, age and gender. *Personality and Mental Health, 11*(1), 37–50.
35. Holzinger, A., Floris, F., Schomerus, G., Carta, M. G., & Angermeyer, M. C. (2012). Gender differences in public beliefs and attitudes about mental disorder in western countries: A systematic review of population studies. *Epidemiology and Psychiatric Sciences, 21*(1), 73–85.
36. Seidler, Z. E., Rice, S. M., Ogrodniczuk, J. S., Oliffe, J. L., & Dhillon, H. M. (2018). Engaging men in psychological treatment: A scoping review. *American Journal of Men's Health, 12*(6), 1882–1900.
37. Gross, J. J., & Levenson, R. W. (1997). Hiding feelings: The acute effects of inhibiting negative and positive emotion. *Journal of Abnormal Psychology, 106*(1), 95–103.
38. Kingston, D., & Tough, S. (2014). Prenatal and postnatal maternal mental health and school-age child development: A systematic review. *Maternal and Child Health Journal, 18*(7), 1728–1741.
39. Brummelte, S., & Galea, L. A. (2016). Postpartum depression: Etiology, treatment and consequences for maternal care. *Hormones and Behavior, 77*, 153–166.
40. Eckenrode, J., Campa, M., Luckey, D. W., Henderson, C. R., Jr., Cole, R., Kitzman, H., Anson, E., Sidora-Arcoleo, K., Powers, J., & Olds, D. (2010). Long-term effects of prenatal and infancy nurse home visitation on the life course of youths: 19-year follow-up of a randomized trial. *Archives of Pediatrics & Adolescent Medicine, 164*(1), 9–15.
41. Orton, L., Pennington, A., Nayak, S., Sowden, A., White, M., & Whitehead, M. (2016). Group-based microfinance for collective empowerment: A systematic review of health impacts. *Bulletin of the World Health Organization, 94*(9), 694–704a.
42. UN. (2015). *The World's Women 2015, Trends and statistics*. https://unstats.un.org/unsd/gender/chapter1/chapter1.html. Accessed 17 Dec 2018.
43. Committee on Ethics. (2015). ACOG Committee Opinion No. 646: Ethical Considerations for Including Women as Research Participants. *Obstetrics and Gynecology, 126*(5), e100–e107.
44. Durant, R. W., Wenzel, J. A., Scarinci, I. C., Paterniti, D. A., Fouad, M. N., Hurd, T. C., & Martin, M. Y. (2014). Perspectives on barriers and facilitators to minority recruitment for clinical trials among cancer center leaders, investigators, research staff, and referring clinicians: Enhancing minority participation in clinical trials (EMPaCT). *Cancer, 120 Suppl 7*, 1097–1105.
45. Lewis, M. E., & Myhra, L. L. (2017). Integrated care with indigenous populations: A systematic review of the literature. *American Indian and Alaska Native Mental Health Research (Online), 24*(3), 88–110.

46. Holden, K., McGregor, B., Thandi, P., Fresh, E., Sheats, K., Belton, A., Mattox, G., & Satcher, D. (2014). Toward culturally centered integrative care for addressing mental health disparities among ethnic minorities. *Psychological Services, 11*(4), 357–368.
47. Benish, S. G., Quintana, S., & Wampold, B. E. (2011). Culturally adapted psychotherapy and the legitimacy of myth: A direct-comparison meta-analysis. *Journal of Counseling Psychology, 58*(3), 279–289.
48. Parra-Cardona, R., Lopez-Zeron, G., Leija, S. G., Maas, M. K., Villa, M., Zamudio, E., Arredondo, M., Yeh, H. H., & Domenech Rodriguez, M. M. (2019). A culturally adapted intervention for Mexican-origin parents of adolescents: The need to overtly address culture and discrimination in evidence-based practice. *Family Process, 58*(2), 334–352.
49. Pan, D., Huey, S. J., Jr., & Hernandez, D. (2011). Culturally adapted versus standard exposure treatment for phobic Asian Americans: Treatment efficacy, moderators, and predictors. *Cultural Diversity & Ethnic Minority Psychology, 17*(1), 11–22.
50. Jenkins, E. K., Kothari, A., Bungay, V., Johnson, J. L., & Oliffe, J. L. (2016). Strengthening population health interventions: Developing the CollaboraKTion framework for community-based knowledge translation. *Health Research Policy and Systems, 14*(1), 65.
51. Jenkins, E. K., Bungay, V., Patterson, A., Saewyc, E. M., & Johnson, J. L. (2018). Assessing the impacts and outcomes of youth driven mental health promotion: A mixed-methods assessment of the Social Networking Action for Resilience study. *Journal of Adolescence, 67*, 1–11.
52. Jagsi, R., Griffith, K. A., Jones, R. D., Stewart, A., & Ubel, P. A. (2017). Factors associated with success of clinician-researchers receiving career development awards from the National Institutes of Health: A Longitudinal Cohort Study. *Academic Medicine: Journal of the Association of American Medical Colleges, 92*(10), 1429–1439.
53. Carnes, M., & Bairey Merz, C. N. (2017). Women are less likely than men to be full professors in cardiology: Why does this happen and how can we fix it? *Circulation, 135*(6), 518–520.
54. Kafer, J., Betancourt, A., Villain, A. S., Fernandez, M., Vignal, C., Marais, G. A. B., & Tenaillon, M. I. (2018). Progress and prospects in gender visibility at SMBE annual meetings. *Genome Biology and Evolution, 10*(3), 901–908.

Chapter 6
Global Mental Health: Services and Access to Care

Priya Ranjan Avinash, Venu Gopal Jhanwar, and Rupali Rohatgi

Key Points
- Mental illness is one of the primary causes of global burden of disease
- Mental health services are often inadequate in developing countries
- Stigma, shame and socio-cultural beliefs are some of the common causes of poor mental health service use
- Certain groups, like cultural and ethnic minorities, women and geriatric population have additional barriers to access health care services
- Gender specific problems in women like post partum disorders and disorders related with menstruation require special attention
- Certain life stages like childhood and old age have their own specific problems, and due to financial, physical and social dependence, this population needs several specific measures to help access to care
- Integration of mental health care to existing primary healthcare is one of the fastest and easiest methods to improve access to care
- Other issues, like stigma, discrimination and prejudice regarding mental illness require remediation measures
- Access to care may be improved using technology, like mobile apps, computers, internet and tele-medicine
- Mental health awareness is lacking in certain communities, and this requires, culture sensitive methods of increasing awareness.
- Globally policy level changes are needed to make mental healthcare at par with general healthcare. These include financial, legislative, infrastructural and human resource measures. Integration of mental healthcare with primary healthcare, separate mental health programs, screening for mental illnesses at community level, protection of rights of people with mental illnesses are some to name a few.

(continued)

P. R. Avinash (✉) · R. Rohatgi
Himalayan Institute of Medical Sciences, Dehradun, India

V. G. Jhanwar
Deva Institute of Healthcare and Research, Varanasi, India

© The Author(s) 2019
S. Bährer-Kohler, B. Bolea-Alamanac (eds.), *Diversity in Global Mental Health*,
SpringerBriefs in Psychology, https://doi.org/10.1007/978-3-030-29112-9_6

- Community mental health services are needed to improve access
- Good mental health where every individual realizes his or her own potential, can cope with the stresses of life, can work productively and fruitfully [1] cannot be achieved, where there is war and poverty. Mental health care delivery requires general economic growth, education, employment in society and above all global peace.

6.1 Introduction

The majority of people suffering from psychological trauma or any life stressors that hamper mental health, lack access to good quality mental health services. Several factors have been proposed which have created a gap in access to mental health services such as social stigma, lack of human resources, segmented delivery of services, lack of knowledge, different policy changes globally, etc. These factors are more prevalent in low and middle income countries [2]. These gaps are more pronounced in women and the transgender population. Also rural and remote areas in the developing world have greater challenges to access to quality mental healthcare.

The Mental Health Gap Action Programme Intervention Guide developed by the World Health Organization (WHO) through its systemic review of evidence followed by consultative participation of several countries has helped to decrease the global mental health (GMH) treatment gap [3]. The WHO Mental Health Gap Action Programme (mhGAP) aims at scaling up services for mental, neurological and substance use disorders especially in countries with low- and middle-incomes. The programme asserts that with proper care, psychosocial assistance and medication, tens of millions could be treated for depression, schizophrenia, and epilepsy, prevented from suicide and begin to lead normal lives– even where resources are scarce [3].

6.2 Content

6.2.1 Diversity, Services and Access to Care

The concept of diversity includes various types of behaviours, culture, ethnicities, religions and environmental and economic influences. For example, in United States, there is a significant rise in individuals from diverse populations due to the number of immigrants entering the country and the increased fertility rate of immigrant populations. Culture also influences different modes of treatment as well as health seeking behaviour, attitudes to providers and expectations about the health care system [4]. There is a vast literature emphasising that health and mental illness are perceived differently across various cultures [5]. This suggest that whether people are motivated to seek treatment, coping strategies, family and community support, where they seek help from a general physician or a registered psychiatrist [6] are all factors that are culturally and socially determined to some extent.

Cultural diversity can also colour perceptions about the aetiology of mental illness. As an example, in Ayurveda (*Ayurveda* is a 5000-year-old system of natural healing that has its origins in the Vedic culture of India), healing from mental illness occurs depending on the karma [refers to the spiritual principle of cause and effect where intent and actions of an individual (cause) influence the future of that individual (effect)] of the subject or one's own actions [7]. It is important to note that people from diverse cultures may not make the same distinction between issues of the body and the mind as in western therapeutic systems. Culture can also affect how people seek treatment as compared to the western health system. Those seeking treatment in India present with more somatic based symptoms as compared with western individuals who tend to present with cognitive based symptoms [8]. Further, research in High Income Countries (HICs) like Australia, Canada and the United States emphasizes that people belonging to diverse cultures in these countries tend to seek help much later than those from non-diverse communities and many of them tend to present in acute stages of mental distress [9].

Hechanova and Waedle suggest that a number of factors related to "shame" explain this low access to mental healthcare [10]. Shame, is defined as a painful feeling of humiliation or distress. The first possibility is the desire to protect the family reputation and their own dignity. The second relates to the possibility that the mental health professional would see them as "crazy," similar to the notion of external shame, and finally that the person may be reluctant to open up to strangers, due to a number of factors such as fears of "loss of face," lack of trust, or the fear of revisiting painful events [10].

Stigma also plays a role in the diversity of treatment seeking behaviours. Stigma can be viewed as a "mark of shame, disgrace or disapproval which results in an individual being rejected, discriminated against, and excluded from participating in a number of different areas of society" [11]. Stigma around depression and other mental illness can be higher in some cultural groups and often is a major barrier to people from diverse cultures when accessing mental health services [9].

Racism and discrimination have significant impact on many cultural groups. Older forms of racism were ideologies that supported the notion of biological "races" and ranked them in terms of superior and inferior, these have been superseded by newer forms of racism that are built on more complex notions of cultural superiority or inferiority [12]. The experience of racism can lead to social alienation of the individual, fear of public spaces, loss of access to services, and a range of other effects that in turn impact adversely on the mental health of the affected individual [9].

Cultural groups can show major differences in terms of the types of stressors that they experience, and how they appraise these stressors [13]. Different cultures may place stressful events as normative, or something that most people in that culture will experience, such as coming-of-age rituals. Further they will allocate social resources in different ways, leading to dissimilar experiences of these stressors. And finally, they may assess stressors differently, such as in terms of breaking of taboos or other cultural norms [13].

How cultural factors impact on the therapeutic relationship is a significant factor to be considered when working with diverse cultures in mental health. In that regard, the provision of the *cultural formulation interview* in the DSM-5 is a positive step especially as it seeks to explore cultural identity, conceptualization of illness, psychosocial stressors, vulnerability, and resilience as well as the cultural features of the relationship between the clinician and the patient [14].

6.2.2   Gender Sensitive Services and Access to Care

Certain mental health disorders are more prevalent in women and play a significant role in the state of women's overall health. The expression of symptoms may also vary by gender or social role. For example, a depressed male would have problems in his job which would be more suggestive of him not going to work and increase in severity and frequency of anger related issues and intake of alcohol whereas a female would complain more of physical symptoms such as fatigability and lethargy and not being able to take care of herself or her family. They are more likely to use religious and emotional outlets to offset the symptoms of depression, especially women in developing countries with poor social and economic background [15]. Women face challenges when it comes to socio- economic power, status and social position. They are still considered to be the primary caregivers for children and elders of their family [15–17]. In many countries women are less empowered due to lesser opportunities of education and respectable employment. Moreover, even those who are financially secure fear crossing social lines and therefore can also be vulnerable. Although the female gender is associated with a favourable outcome for certain mental illnesses like schizophrenia, social consequences such as marital abandonment, homelessness, vulnerability to sexual abuse, and subsequent exposure to HIV and other infections contribute to the difficulties of the rehabilitation of women. The prevalence rates for sexual and physical abuse of women with severe mental illnesses are twice those observed in the general population of women. In India, the absence of any clear policies for the welfare of severely ill women, and the social stigma further compounds the problem [18] adding to the lack of gender sensitive mental health services.

However, in contrast to the data from many other countries, women outnumber men in completed suicides in India [19]. Biswas et al., found that girls from nuclear families and women married at a very young age to be at a higher risk for attempted suicide and self-harm. The suicide rate by age for India reveals that suicide rates peak for both men and women between the age 18 and 29 while in the age group 10–17, the rate in females exceeds the male fig [20].

According to an eye-opening United Nations report published in 2005, around two-third of married women in India are victims of domestic violence and each incident of violence translated into women losing 7 working days in the country. Furthermore, as many as 70% of married women between the ages of 15 and 49 years have been subjected to physical violence, sexual assault or coerced sex [21]. Countries like India, where the family system is still predominantly "joint type" (conventional or traditional patriarchal family system, where a man, his wife, their children stay with man's other brother(s) and their family including the living parents of the man live together in a house, with the head of the family being the man's father), the roles and responsibility of women puts them at increased risk of mental illness and burnout. The consequences of gender based differences include lifelong mental and emotional distress, post traumatic stress disorder (PTSD) and poor reproductive health [22].

In India, postpartum blues affect 50–80% of mothers [23]. Low income, birth of a daughter when a son was desired, relationship difficulties with relatives, adverse life events during pregnancy and lack of physical help are all risk factors reported in Indian women for the onset of postpartum depression. In addition, the postpartum period carries the potential for exacerbation of psychiatric symptoms in women with pre-existing mental illness [24]. Furthermore, when a woman becomes mentally ill, services are sought infrequently and late. Rather she is blamed for the illness. She may be socially ostracized or abandoned by her husband and her own family. Hence, being a "woman" and being "mentally ill" is perceived as a dual 'curse'. Even though some authors feel that marriage protects against psychological breakdown, this is not always the case. Several studies show that there is greater distress in married women as compared to married men. The birth of a child, abortion or miscarriage, economic stresses, and major career changes are some of the stressful events in married life some of which are gender specific [25].

Greater stigma is attached to women's mental illness which restricts the use of public health services and lessens the importance of mental wellbeing in women's health [26]. Education, specific training, and interventions targeting the social and physical environment are crucial for addressing women's mental health needs. Identification of significant persons in government departments and other relevant groups in the community, to obtain and document data indicating the extent of women's problems and the burden associated with women's mental health problems and the development of policies to protect and promote women's mental health are extremely crucial.

Services should be implemented at primary care delivery as well as on legal and judicial fronts. Good quality mental health services should be available at the primary care level. Primary care providers must be aware of the major mental health problems affecting women, routinely enquire about common mental health problems, provide the most appropriate intervention and support and provide education to the community on issues related to the mental health of women. The financial dependence of many women along with the societal role expectations specially lead to decrease help seeking when a mental health problem arises. Mental health care needs to be integrated with reproductive health as both cannot be considered separately from each other.

6.2.3   Access to Mental Health Care for Transgender Individuals

Transgender individuals suffer from direct barriers to access health care, including lack of insurance coverage along with indirect barriers such as unfriendly social environments and perceived stigma for both the patients themselves and the providers of transgender health care [27]. Individuals who identify as transgender tend to experience higher rates of mental health issues than the general population. According to a study published in 2016 "distress and impairment, considered essential characteristics of mental disorders" among transgender individuals primarily arises in response to the discrimination, stigma, lack of acceptance, and abuse they face on an unfortunately regular basis [28]. Stigma can also directly affect health by encouraging ostracized individuals to avoid social encounters, shy away from healthcare professionals, reach for addictive substances to quell their anxiety and isolation, or engage in risk-taking behaviours, like unsafe sex. Mental health disparity is largely due to transphobia, gender related discrimination and abuse [29]. There is a need to have provisions for exclusive mental health services addressing the specific needs of the transexual population.

6.2.4   Access to Care Across the Lifespan

6.2.4.1   Childhood

Mental health problems are common and typically have an early onset. Even where effective treatments for mental health problems in childhood and adolescence are available, yet only a minority of children who are affected access them. This is a serious concern, considering the far-reaching and long-term negative consequences of such problems. Primary care is usually the first port of call for concerned parents so it is important to understand how primary care practitioners manage child and adolescent mental health problems and the challenges they face [30]. Primary care practitioners play a crucial 'gatekeeper' role to specialist services for children and young people with mental health problems, yet they face numerous barriers, in particular a lack of clinical time, knowledge, reimbursement, access to specialized mental health providers, and resources. A study done in the US in 2000 concludes that lack of providers of specialist services was the most highly endorsed barrier overall, with primary care practitioners expressing a clear desire for decreased waiting times and increased resources for referral, particularly in rural areas [31].

Some families are unable to access care due to shortage of child psychiatrists, psychologists and behaviour therapists or unavailability of any care in the vicinity. Telemedicine can be useful to fill these gaps in care [32]. Mental health and primary health care can work together to include mental and behavioural health screening and treatment into primary care. This approach is commonly known as behavioural health integration.

6.2.4.2   Older Age

Another life stage that puts excessive burden on mental and emotional health is the old age. Disparity in access to health care among elderly Americans has been well documented [33]. Ageism is quite prevalent in most societies, more so in the western world. People in the geriatric age group have many co-morbid medical illnesses, adding a financial burden, along with reduced earnings, compounded by lack of social support and loneliness. All these factors contribute to mental illness, and bring unique challenges to its treatment. Psychological and physical barriers affect access to care among the elderly; these may be influenced by poverty more than by race [34]. Older people in particular have been found to dislike having to seek referral to specialist services from family doctors [35]. It has also been suggested that sociodemographic factors (such as educational, economical, regional, ethical and cultural factors) also result in reduced access to healthcare for older people [36]. Many older people may not have caregivers, either due to death or separation, or have caregivers who are old themselves, further contributing to gap in access to health care services. Older people usually many chronic medical illness, which requires intensive care management and reduces their mobility, leading to poor access to mental health care facilities [37].

6.3   Discussion

6.3.1   Ideas and Development, Evidence and Recommendation Guidelines

It has been observed that one of the biggest gaps in access to mental healthcare is lack of knowledge. This is more so in the developing countries. This lack of knowledge regarding mental illnesses combined with various stigmas associated with mental illness lead to poor access to mental healthcare facilities. Educational programs using methods like, pamphlets, radio programs, television advertisements, billboards, street plays etc. specially in the language and context familiar to the community, would be most useful. In many countries where primary healthcare services are well developed, the existing health care workers can be entrusted with dissemination of knowledge to the leaders of the communities without any extra cost or burden.

Among many approaches to improve access to services there has been recent focus on novel systems for the delivery of interventions. By delivering a service in a primary health centre or community health centre or by using non traditional methods of service delivery, for example through the help of telemedicine techniques, the access to care gap can be filled [38, 39]. Also the nature of interventions both pharmacological as well as non-pharmacological ones can be modified in tune with the cultural beliefs or presentations of a disorder within a particular ethnic group [40, 41].

6.3.2   The Recommendations to Improve the Global Mental Health Care Access Can Be Summarized As

- Educate the community about the various mental health problems
- Use community specific models, keeping the social and cultural background into account while disseminating information regarding mental health
- Use of various novel methods for education, like media, internet, charts, posters, films, radio and TV programs etc.
- Integrate mental healthcare with existing primary healthcare services
- Seek cooperation and active participation of community leaders like teachers, local political leaders, preachers, informal community health workers etc.
- Use telemedicine to provide specialist services in remote areas
- Provide cheaper and effective methods of treatment, to help maintenance on long term treatment, as compliance is of utmost importance in case of mental healthcare.
- Special focus should be for socially weaker groups including: cultural and ethnic minorities, women, children, geriatric population and sexual minorities

6.4   Brief Conclusion

Global mental health's biggest challenges are lack of adequate mental health care services and various barriers to access of care. These barriers are gender, lifespan and social and cultural group specific. Policy level decisions at the top and administrative priority to mental health services at the grass root level can help amend many of these barriers. Awareness programs in the communities own language can help reduce stigma and facilitate seeking of modern mental healthcare even among societies traditionally known to shun them. Integrating existing primary health care services with mental health services is probably one of the most economical and effective methods for providing quality accessible mental health care to all. Telemedicine technologies can help achieve the same goals in areas where specialists are scarce [32].

Future Tasks

To improve mental healthcare access globally, there are certain tasks which need to be undertaken on a priority basis, in future.

- Develop a consensus on "there is no health without mental health"
- Launch a common minimum program for mental health, globally
- Policy and global funding for "mental health for all" need to be taken as a priority by UN and WHO

- Thorough assessment of local needs and local conditions, is required to formulate a tailor made program for each community
- Special Focus on minority and vulnerable populations, like women, children, old age, LGBT community and ethnic and religious minorities
- Integrate mental healthcare with primary healthcare
- Both generalist and specialist assessment and intervention services in primary care settings
- Develop man-power by increasing the number of specialists, like psychiatrists, clinical psychologists, psychiatric social workers and psychiatric nurses.
- Use existing technology (for example, text messages, email, telephone, computers, mobile apps, virtual reality etc) for people who may find it difficult to, or choose not to, attend a specific service and Tele-mental health for remote areas
- Develop newer technologies for improving access to care.

References

1. WHO. (2014). *Mental health: A state of well-being.* https://www.who.int/features/factfiles/mental_health/en/. Retrieved 29 Jan 2019.
2. Wainberg, M. L., et al. (2017). Challenges and opportunities in global mental health: A research-to-practice perspective. *Current Psychiatry Reports, 19*(5), 28.
3. WHO. (2016). *MHGAP intervention guide for mental, neurological and substance use disorders in nonspecialized health settings version 2.0.* Geneva: World Health Organization.
4. Gopalkrishnan, N. (2014). Integrative medicine and mental health: Implications for social work practice. In A. Francis (Ed.), *Social work practice in mental health: Theories, practices and challenges.* New Delhi: Sage Publications.
5. Fernando, S. (2015). *Race and culture in psychiatry.* Hove: Routledge.
6. Office of the Surgeon General (US); Center for Mental Health Services (US); National Institute of Mental Health (US). Mental Health. (2001). Culture, race, and ethnicity: A supplement to mental health: A report of the surgeon general. Rockville, MD: Substance Abuse and Mental Health Services Administration (US). Available from: https://www.ncbi.nlm.nih.gov/books/NBK44243/.
7. Kirmayer, L. J. (2004). The cultural diversity of healing: Meaning, metaphor and mechanism. *British Medical Bulletin, 16*, 33–48.
8. Biswas, J., Gangadhar, B. N., & Keshavan, M. (2016). Cross cultural variations in psychiatrists' perception of mental illness: A tool for teaching culture in psychiatry. *Asian Journal of Psychiatry, 23*, 1–7.
9. FECCA. (2011). *Mental health and Australia's culturally and linguistically diverse communities: A submission to the senate standing committee on community affairs.* Canberra: The Federation of Ethnic Communities' Councils of Australia.
10. Hechanova, M. R. M., Tuliao, A. P., Teh, L. A., Jr., & Acosta, A. (2013). Problem severity, technology adoption, and intent to seek online counseling among overseas filipino workers. *Cyberpsychology, Behavior, and Social Networking, 16*, 613–617.
11. WHO The World Health Report 2001. (2001). *Mental health: New understanding, new hope.* Geneva: World Health Organization.

12. Babacan, H., & Gopalkrishnan, N. (2007). *Racisms in the New World order: Realities of culture, colour and identity.* Newcastle: Cambridge Scholars Publishing.
13. Aldwin, C. M. (2004). *Culture, coping and resilience to stress.* In: Paper Presented at the First International Conference on Operationalization of Gross National Happiness, Thimphu.
14. Ang, W. (2017). Bridging culture and psychopathology in mental health care. *European Child and Adolescent Psychiatry, 26*, 263–266.
15. Shidhaye, R., & Patel, V. (2010). Association of socio-economic, gender and health factors with common mental disorders in women: A population-based study of 5703 married rural women in India. *International Journal of Epidemiology, 39*, 1510–1521.
16. Debra B lyn Hook, common mental health issues in women (2012).
17. Eaton, N. R., Keyes, K. M., Krueger, R. F., Balsis, S., Skodol, A. E., Markon, K. E., et al. (2012). An invariant dimensional liability model of gender differences in mental disorder prevalence: Evidence from a national sample. *Journal of Abnormal Psychology, 121*, 282–288.
18. Thara, R., & Patel, V. (2001). Women's mental health: A public health concern. In *Regional health forum-WHO South-East Asia Region* (Vol. 5, pp. 24–34). World Health Organization.
19. Rao, V. (2004). Suicidology: The Indian context. In S. P. Agarwal (Ed.), *Mental health: An Indian perspective 1946–2003* (pp. 279–284). New Delhi: Directorate General of Health Services/Ministry of Health and Family Welfare Nirman Bhawan.
20. Biswas, S., Roy, S., Debnath, C., & Sengupta, S. B. (1997). A study of attempted suicide in adolescents in West Bengal. *Indian Journal of Psychiatry, 39*, 54–55.
21. Press Trust of India. (2005). *Two-third married Indian women victims of domestic violence: UN.* Posted Online; Thursday, October 13.
22. Gomel, M. K. (1997). *A focus on women.* Geneva: World Health Organization.
23. Chandra, P. S., Carey, M. P., Carey, K. B., Shalinianant, A., & Thomas, T. (2003). Sexual coercion and abuse among women with a severe mental illness in India: An exploratory investigation. *Comprehensive Psychiatry, 44*, 205–212.
24. Chandran, M., Tharyan, P., Muliyil, J., & Abraham, S. (2002). Post-partum depression in a cohort of women from a rural area of Tamil Nadu, India. Incidence and risk factors. *The British Journal of Psychiatry, 181*, 499–504.
25. Nambi, S. (2005). *Marriage, mental health and INDIAN legislation.* 57th Annual National Conference of the Indian Psychiatric Society. Chandigarh.
26. Sood, A. (2008). *Women's pathways to mental health in India.* UC Los Angeles: UCLA Center for the Study of Women.
27. Safer, J. D., et al. (2016). Barriers to healthcare for transgender individuals. *Current Opinion in Endocrinology, Diabetes, and Obesity, 23*(2), 168–171.
28. Robles, R., Fresán, A., Vega-Ramirez, H., et al. (2016). Removing transgender identity from the classification of mental disorders: A Mexican field study for ICD-11. *The Lancet, 3*(9), 850–859.
29. MIzock, L. Transgender and gender diverse clients with mental disorders. *Psychiatry Clinics, 40*(1), 29–30.
30. O'Brien, D., et al. (2016). Barriers to managing child and adolescent mental health problems: A systematic review of primary care practitioners' perceptions. *British Journal of General Practice, 66,651*, e693–e707.
31. Briggs-Gowan, M. J., Horwitz, S. M., Schwab-Stone, M. E., et al. (2000). Mental health in pediatric settings: Distribution of disorders and factors related to service use. *Journal of the American Academy of Child and Adolescent Psychiatry, 39*(7), 841–849.
32. Langarizadeh, M., Tabatabaei, M. S., Tavakol, K., Naghipour, M., Rostami, A., & Moghbeli, F. (2017). Telemental health care, an effective alternative to conventional mental care: A systematic review. *Actainformaticamedica: AIM: journal of the Society for Medical Informatics of Bosnia & Herzegovina: casopis DrustvazamedicinskuinformatikuBiH, 25*(4), 240–246.
33. McCormick, M. C., Weinick, R. M., Elixhauser, A., Stagnitti, M. N., Thompson, J., & Simpson, I. (2001). Annual report on access to and utilization of health care for children and youth in the United States–2000. *Ambulatory Pediatrics, 1*, 3–15.

34. Fitzpatrick, A. L., et al. (2004). Barriers to health care access among the elderly and who perceives them. *American Journal of Public Health, 94*(10), 1788–1794.
35. Dixon-Woods, M., Kirk, D., Agarwal, S., et al. (2005). *Vulnerable groups and access to health care: A critical interpretive review*. London: National Co-ordinating Centre for NHS Service Delivery and Organisation. [10 August 2011]. Report for the National Co-ordinating Centre for NHS Service Delivery and Organisation R & D (NCCSDO) Available at: http://www.sdo.nihr.ac.uk/files/project/SDO_ES_08-1210-025_V01.pdf.
36. Chaix, B., Merlo, J., & Chauvin, P. (2005). Comparison of a spatial approach with the multilevel approach for investigating place effects on health: The example of healthcare utilisation in France. *Journal of Epidemiology and Community Health., 59*, 517–526.
37. WHO. (2017). *Mental health: fact sheet*. https://www.who.int/news-room/fact-sheets/detail/mental-health-of-older-adults/. Retrieved on 08 Feb 2019.
38. Powell, J. (2002). Systematic review of outreach clinics in primary care in the UK. *Journal of Health Services Research and Policy, 7*, 177–178.
39. Gulliford, M., Figueroa-Munoz, J., Morgan, M., et al. (2007). What does 'access to health care' mean? *Journal of Health Services Research & Policy., 7*, 186–188.
40. Bernal, G., & Domenech Rodriguez, M. M. (2009). Advances in Latino family research: Cultural adaptations of evidence-based interventions. *Family Process, 48*, 169–178.
41. National Collaborating Centre for Mental Health (UK). (2011). *Common mental health disorders: Identification and pathway to care NICE Clinical Guidelines, No. 123*. Leicester (UK): British Psychological Society.

Chapter 7
Mental Health/Global Mental Health: Prevention and Promotion with the Inclusion of Diversity and Gender – A Binational Integration Initiative

Monica Chavira and Lucia Durá

Key Points
- Prevention and Promotion of mental health are very important in order to reduce the heavy burden of mental and physical disorders.
- This chapter presents a brief overview of mental health disparities in access to care in the U.S.-Mexico border. It presents unique life stressors that border and migrant populations face can become risk factors for developing mental illness.
- The first section points out measures aimed at strengthening the gender and cultural perspective in the promotion of mental health and prevention of illness by training community health workers that can help reduce gaps in inequalities and the risk of developing mental illness.
- The second section offers a summary of *The Mental Health Gap Action Program (mhGAP) from the World Health Organization* that was used as a framework for the initiative in the border states. MhGAP has been widely used worldwide and in different American countries successfully, and a pilot version tailored to Community Health Workers (CHW) was used for the first time.
- The third section provides the highlights of a case study of the two border communities piloting the mhGAP for CHW's, and how integration of mental health into primary health care reduces burden of mental illness, and promotes holistic care.

(continued)

M. Chavira, MA (✉) · L. Durá, PhD
The University of Texas at El Paso, El Paso, United States
e-mail: chaviram@miners.utep.edu

© The Author(s) 2019
S. Bährer-Kohler, B. Bolea-Alamanac (eds.), *Diversity in Global Mental Health*,
SpringerBriefs in Psychology, https://doi.org/10.1007/978-3-030-29112-9_7

- The fourth section presents a discussion on how community health workers can be part of the referral system for primary health care to increase wellbeing and resilience across the life span.
- Finally, the last part of the chapter provides future tasks in a bicultural scenario where access to care takes into account gender and cultural differences that promote access to care, self-care strategies and reduction of stigma.

7.1 Introduction

Mental illness prevention and mental health promotion are important steps in the reduction of the burden of mental and physical disorders [19]. Epidemiological reports of prevalence rates indicate that worldwide 1 in 5 people experience a mental health condition with 300 million people suffering from depression alone [39]. In the US-Mexico border region, suicide rates accounted for 12.1 per 100,000 deaths in the US [8, 9] and 4.2 per 100,000 in Mexico [1, 20]. These border populations face stressors that place them at a higher risk to develop mental health disorders: immigration, grieving, health disparities and barriers to health care.

Training community health workers (CHW) in mental health is a cost-effective and evidence-based intervention which can (1) reduce the burden of mental disorders, (2) provide greater access to care for all, (3) reduce stigma, (4) treat comorbid mental and physical illnesses and (5) increase human rights vigilance.

The present case study focuses on the integration of mental health into primary health through the Mental Health Gap Action Program (mhGAP) [14], a model of care that incorporates CHW in mental health promotion and mental illness [15]. It illustrates the experiences of a binational mhGAP-CHW integration program on the US-Mexico border, a region with notable disparities: the US, a high-income country (HIC) and Mexico a low-income country (LIC).

7.2 Content

7.2.1 Mental Health/Global Mental Health: Prevention and Promotion with the Inclusion of Diversity and Gender

To provide an integral scope of mental health and its social determinants, this section provides an overview of how CHWs can help with promotion of mental health and well-being and prevention of illness to reduce gender and diversity inequalities [6, 18]. As migrant populations increase in a globalized world, so does cultural diversity, which has an impact on mental health. The US-Mexico border is an example of this phenomena. CHWs that are underutilizing of mental health services by vulnerable populations [16], and differences in perceived need may contribute to these disparities [7].

One of the most vulnerable populations are migrants and refugees who are at a higher risk of developing a mental illness because of the trauma they suffered during their migration journey or in their native countries [27]. Minority populations that are common in border areas also face a constellation of life stressors that may have unique influences on mental illness and how it is perceived: including discrimination and segregation that can make them afraid of using mental health services [28–30]. Evidence shows that many people in culturally and linguistically diverse populations have co-morbidity issues, poor self-management of chronic illness and reluctance to seek mental and disability support services [4, 31, 32].

CHWs are perceived as allies, since they are part of the community and can help remove structural barriers as well as provide information and follow up in cases where no other access to services is possible [12]. Thus, CHWs can play a critical role in supporting community-based services and teams in early intervention, well-being and recovery [10, 13]. Since on the US-Mexico border many CHWs are bilingual and speak the native language of many migrants, the aspects of language barrier are mitigated or disappear. CHWs can help in influencing help-seeking behavior by reducing stigma, promoting mental health and changing perceived need, i.e., the misconception a person may have regarding their own mental health as good, when in reality they may be experiencing a mental health condition.

In healthcare, a gender perspective can help us identify the different treatment needs and venues to reduce stigma and inequalities for access to services which can be applied to mental health [5]. For example, women tend to express their feelings more often with their peers and seek help compared to men [8]. In contrast, men may have negative perceptions towards needing and seeking services in mental health, due to western masculine norms [33]. Women are also more susceptible to psychosocial stressors than men [11]. Incorporating the gender and diversity perspective in the promotion and prevention of mental health is an essential aspect to reduce disparities in mental health services utilization [14, 34].

7.3   The mhGAP Approach and Integration of Mental Health into Primary Health Care

In 2008 the World Health Organization (WHO) launched mhGAP worldwide in order to scale services for mental, neurological and substance use disorders through the integration of mental health into primary care [14, 20–22].

In the Americas, mhGAP was first introduced in 2010 [14] in Panama and in 2011 on the Mexican border city of Juárez. Experts from the WHO investigated key elements to integrate mental health into primary health care, including evidence-based practices in 11 different countries around the world. Several advantages for the integration were noted [23]: the burden of mental disorders, the treatment gap, the interrelation between mental and physical health and improvement of overall patient health through holistic treatment. Other benefits are the reduction of stigma and access to care, as services are anchored in the community and allow monitoring, while respecting the privacy of individuals and their human rights. Additionally, integration is cost effective and it can be implemented in LICs (*low*-income countries) and MICs (*middle*-income countries) [23].

In a study that compared the expected average annual cost of treating the different priority disorders in a non-specialist healthcare setting using the mhGAP intervention guide in five countries, was ranging between $0.21 and $1.86 per capita [35]. The costs are also lower for the main care givers that suffer harsh economic impacts need including lost days of work, travelling time to the clinics and expenses [36].

The mhGAP strategy begins with a needs assessment, followed with a "train the trainers program" that provides CHW (community health workers) personnel with the tools to identify and refer patients with 11 priority conditions: depression, psychosis, bipolar disorder, epilepsy and seizures, child and adolescent mental disorders, dementia, stress disorders, developmental disorders, alcohol abuse and substance use disorders. CHW personnel may refer patients with other conditions as well, but the above are prioritized.

The pyramid in Fig. 7.1 represents the mhGAP model of care [24]. At the first two levels of the pyramid, CHW roles entail promotion of self-care and mental health prevention as well as referring people to mental health services or to mental health care at the primary care level.

The primary role of a CWH is to serve as an advocate for the well-being of others in the community. It is important to note that CHWs tend to be female volunteers who are recruited via non-profit organizations or local healthcare providers. The types of people who might fit into this role could include, but are not limited to interested and responsible neighbors, church volunteers, case managers and outreach workers. CHWs aim to promote emotional and mental health well-being, promoting daily mental hygiene. The CHW may facilitate access to medical care and

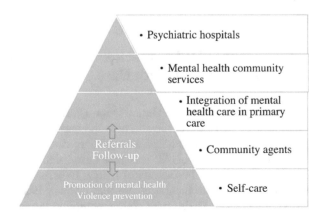

Fig. 7.1 The role of community health workers trained in mental health. (Adapted from: World Health Organization [18, 19])

serve as a liaison between the care provider and community member, observing progress and providing feedback, while promoting individual empowerment by inspiring their peers (most CHWs are women) to continue their education, manage their finances responsibly and work to build their confidence. CHWs can motivate change in their peers, increase awareness in mental health and well-being and reduce stigma in their communities. Thus, incorporating CHWs into the integration of mental health and primary health care (PHC) on the US-Mexico border seemed like a natural strategy. It promotes a mechanism for networking, collaboration and information exchange, enabling CHWs and PHC personnel to work together systemically to leverage resources and service delivery [2].

Various systematic reviews and studies have shown evidence that the integration of CHWs into a collaborative model of care works. Braun [37] stressed the significance of CHWs as a bridge between the community and the health system, as well as an entry point to provide access to "hard to reach populations." Another key element is the importance of mobile technology in their delivery of health services. A study using mobile phones in a pilot study with 75 CHW in Malawi showed improvement in time efficiency. The savings in time increased the CHW's work capacity, in a course of 6 months they saved 2048 hours of work and spent $2750 less in fuel and other related work costs, which gave them the opportunity to treat the double number of clients. Another outcome of using mobile technology is in the positive association with confidence in their abilities and higher self-efficacy (.25, $p < .001$), as shown in the Aceh-Bhear study [37].

Padmanathan and De Silva [16] also found that the incorporation of CHWs in the front lines has helped to identify people with mental illnesses and refer them to providers or find emergency counseling.

Kok [38] explored the intermediate position of the community health workers (CHWs) between the health system and the community. In terms of the relationship between the CHWs and the health sector, all countries showed a formalized support system that included supervision and training [38]. One program from Mozambique had specific protocols with supervision at the district and health facility level. Supervisors were assigned a CHW group from a health facility and provide CHWs with checklists to report on their work duties, referrals, and the collection of drug and supply kits from health facilities [12].

Research shows evidence of CHWs as an effective human resource in addressing physical health disparities, but few studies CHW's impact on mental health interventions. Barnett et al. [3] examined 43 articles to understand the efforts of CHWs in delivering evidence-based mental health interventions to populations that are hard to reach in the US. These interventions delivered by CHWs can be categorized in three sections:

- outreach,
- promotion and management and
- following up adherence to treatment.

CHW inclusion in the mhGAP pyramid of services expands human resource capacity, lowers costs and increases access to care according to previous evidence-based WHO interventions to integrate mental health. The preliminary data from the state of

Chihuahua, Mexico showed the capacity to treat mental health disorders by primary health care physicians trained in mhGAP increased by 55% from 2014 to 2015, and the referrals provided by CHWs to Primary Health Care personnel were 3065 [15].

7.4 US-Mexico Border Case Study

The binational integration initiative where the first mhGAP cohort was trained was carried out in Ciudad Juárez, México, from 2010 to 2013. This training was followed by two cohorts in the Mexican cities of Tijuana, Baja California and Nogales, Sonora. Following that initial project, the Panamerican Health Organization (PAHO) was approached by the Border Health Commission in the US to explore the possibility of running a similar project on the American side of the border [15].

The project then grew to implement similar components in a designated set of border city communities. A situational analysis using the WHO Assessment Instrument for Mental Health Systems (AIMS) and telephone interviews were conducted to assess local priorities in four pairs of cities across the border: Ciudad Juárez-El Paso, Tijuana-San Diego, Laredo-Nuevo Laredo and Reynosa- McAllen. The analysis showed substantial health system challenges in mental health across the cities including insufficient resources of mental health professionals, lack of primary health care personnel trained in mental health and deficient information systems. [15]. The three priority conditions identified and shared across the cities were depression, anxiety disorders and substance abuse. Based on the situational analysis, it was highly recommended to invest resources into training professionals and CHWs about mental health issues. By giving them adequate skills and knowledge, the existing short-staffed mental health workforce could then be expanded.

An implementation alliance was established between the following organizations to fund the initiative: PAHO in the US; the US Substance Abuse and Mental Health Services Administration (SAMHSA); the US Department of Health and Human Services; the Secretary of Health (Mexican Ministry of Health) and the National Commission for Mental Health (CONSAME, acronym in Spanish) in Mexico; and the Border Health Commission in both countries.

7.5 Methodology

The mhGAP for CHW training was coordinated by the state on the Mexico side and by the cities or counties on the US side. An adaptation meeting with a group of experts from each region took place before implementation. Monitoring and evaluation used the mhGAP monitoring and evaluation toolkit that included the following resources adapted for this project:

- Training evaluation forms (from the mhGAP Course Planning Guide);
- Mental, neurological and substance use patient visit summary; and
- Pre-and Post-Test for PHC personnel and CHW.

Focus groups and individual interviews using mhGAP monitoring and evaluation tools were conducted both face to face and via webinar to understand satisfaction and attitudes about Mental, Neurological and Substance Use disorders as well as changes in perceptions that took place with follow up meetings. The use of technological apps (specifically, WhatsApp) allowed for the creation of four groups to share experiences, questions and material related to mental health. A series of indicators and preliminary results from two counties of the state of Chihuahua, where the first mhGAP cohort was trained, included the number of referrals to specialist care and the number of people trained in mhGAP.

- In the US, 270 community health workers from 9 cities in 4 border states (Texas, New Mexico, Arizona and California) were trained in mhGAP. From the 270 trainees, only 23 were male. The majority of the male CHW's belonged to a group called BETA that treats immigrant populations [11].
- In the Mexican states, a total of 1585 community health workers (only 2% were male) were trained from the cities of Tijuana, Palomas, Ciudad Juarez, Ojinaga, Reynosa, Matamoros and Nuevo Laredo. The training and supervision of trainees was provided by a mental health consultant hired by PAHO.

Follow up sessions with CHWs trained during the period of 2014–2015 were initially contemplated via webinars and face to face refresher courses that included a Psychological First Aid (PFA) for field workers for CHWs from the cities of Juarez, Mexico, El Paso, Texas and Las Cruces, New Mexico. In the training participants learned the core skills of observing, listening to and referring distressed people.

The capacity development for CHWs was ensured by the following elements:

- Alignment of the role of CHWs through inter-sectoral coordination and synergy between the community and the greater health system (represented by the Secretary of Health and Health and Human Services).
- 12-hour initial training consisting of eight modules of competency-based training, theory and role play practices.

One of the successes of the intervention rested in the appropriate recruitment and selection of providers on both sides of the border thanks to the leadership of the Border Health Commission, the Department of Health and Human Services, and Texas Tech School of Medicine in the US as well as the Ministry of Health in Mexico (Comision Binacional Fronteriza 2017; [15]). The CHWs trained performed outreach, promotion and management, following up on adherence to treatment.

7.6 Discussion

There are many challenges and opportunities to integrating mental health into primary health care in border regions, especially where health disparities abound. The differences in health care systems and insurance companies in the US prevent full adoption of the mhGAP model, as there exist a wide variety of health care provisions without a unified system. In the case of Mexico, the mhGAP model has been adopted promptly as the CONSAME (National Council of Mental Health) has made it part of their integration strategy in all 32 states including the 6 border states. A key element of the adaptation lies in the incorporation of the Autonomous University of Mexico (known in Spanish as UNAM) that has begun a training program for trainers: mainly psychiatrists, primary care physicians, nurses and psychologists to train primary health care personnel in the 11 priority conditions of the mhGAP.

Another issue surrounding integration is that the role that gender and diversity play, which may put specific populations at risk is not always taken into account. Measures aimed at strengthening the gender and cultural perspective in CHWs are advisable and the incorporation of more male CHWs as it will help destigmatize mental health and reduce inequalities. Male CHWs were scarce in the training, accounting for only 2% of the total of CHWs and this limits the possibility of male clients feeling comfortable approaching CHWs and seeking help. It is paramount to understand how gender inequality and inequalities in access to resources influences mental illness.

In order to overcome these challenges and make a strategy successful certain elements need to be in place. An initial mental health assessment in the country or region where integration will take place is needed to provide a clear panoramic picture of the mental health situation. Such an assessment should deliberately consider gender differences as well as ethnic and linguistic needs to provide multiculturally diverse and locally relevant services. This mental health assessment would first investigate the existing structures of how providers work within the different sectors, the primary, secondary and tertiary, what insurance policies (such as Medicare and Medicaid) cover behavioral health and what the existing budget allocated by the local, state and federal governments is. Secondly, the assessment would include human resources including the PHC- CHW who are trained in mental health and the availability of psychotropic medication for priority conditions such as depression, anxiety disorders, psychosis, dementia, epilepsy, developmental disorders and conduct disorders. Thirdly, a careful monitoring and evaluation system should be placed to record mental health data, understand the prevalence of disorders and devise strategies to approach future treatment.

7.7   Brief Conclusion

This case study from the US-Mexico border depicts what a critical role CHWs have in mental health systems, from promotion and prevention strategies to referral and follow up activities. Although all groups of trained CHWs conducted mental health and wellbeing support activities, through cultural awareness days and other commemorative events, not every group was able to systematize their experience due to the lack of formal training. Some of the most prominent events were organized through WhatsApp, such as World Mental Health Day which was a binational initiative. Critical gaps identified were the lack of continuous funding and supervision, as well as tracking all promotion and prevention activities by the CHW's in the ten border states.

Future Tasks

- Given the growing burden of mental disorders, it is essential that effective preventive and promotional interventions are offered and integrated to reduce the impact of mental disorders on individuals and societies [26].
- The importance of the role of the CHWs within the formal public health system, cannot be underestimated, CHWs can play a crucial role in supporting the primary health care services in early detection, promotion of wellbeing and follow up for patients in adherence to treatment.
- There is a need to establish paid personnel positions for CHWs, particularly in LIC countries, where the role is primarily volunteer-based and prevents them from being a part of a formal referral system.
- CHWs should also be trained in community assessment, as they can be an asset in identifying needs and barriers to care as well as in designing and planning integrated care actions for the community.

References

1. Atlas Country Resources for Neurological Disorders. Retrieved on 19 Sept 2017 from: http://apps.who.int/iris/bitstream/10665/258947/1/9789241565509-eng.pdf. One additional resource of student's choice.
2. Abdulmalik, J., & Thornicroft, G. (2016). Community mental health: A brief, global perspective. *Neurology, Psychiatry and Brain Research, 22*, 101–104. https://doi.org/10.1016/j.npbr.2015.12.065.
3. Barnett, M. L., Gonzalez, A., Miranda, J., Chavira, D. A., & Lau, A. S. (2017). Mobilizing community health workers to address mental health disparities for underserved populations: A systematic review. *Administration and Policy in Mental Health and Mental Health Services Research*, 1–17.
4. Corrigan, P. W., Druss, B. G., & Perlick, D. A. (2014). The impact of mental illness stigma on seeking and participating in mental health care. *Psychological Science in the Public Interest, 15*(2), 37–70.
5. Dedovic, K., Wadiwalla, M., Engert, V., & Pruessner, J. C. (2009). The role of sex and gender socialization in stress reactivity. *Developmental Psychology, 45*, 45–55.
6. Francis, A. P., Pulla, V., & Goel, K. (2014). Community development and mental health promotion. In K. Goel, V. Pulla, & A. P. Francis (Eds.), *Community work: Theories, experiences and challenges* (pp. 162–180). Bangalore: Niruta Publications.
7. Hernandez, M., Nesman, T., Mowery, D., Acevedo-Polakovich, I. D., & Callejas, L. M. (2009). Cultural competence: A literature review and conceptual model for mental health services. *Psychiatric Services, 60*, 1046–1050. https://doi.org/10.1176/ps.2009.60.8.1046.
8. Jorm, A. F. (2000). Mental health literacy: Public knowledge and beliefs about mental disorders. *British Journal of Psychiatry, 177*(5), 396–401.

9. Juster, R. P., Pruessner, J. C., Desrochers, A. B., Bourdon, O., Durand, N., Wan, N., et al. (2016). Sex and gender roles in relation to mental health and allostatic load. *Psychosomatic Medicine, 78*(7), 788–804.
10. Mental Health America. (2016, October 17). Retrieved 15 Sept 2017 from http://www.mentalhealthamerica.net/issues/state-mental-health-america
11. Meyer, I. H. (2015). Resilience in the study of minority stress and health of sexual and gender minorities. *Psychology of Sexual Orientation and Gender Diversity, 2*(3), 209–213.
12. Ndima, S. D., Sidat, M., Give, C., Ormel, H., Kok, M. C., & Taegtmeyer, M. (2015). Supervision of community health workers in Mozambique: A qualitative study of factors influencing motivation and programme implementation. *Human Resources for Health, 13*(1), 63.
13. Lando, J., Williams, S. M., Williams, B., & Sturgis, S. (2006). A logic model for the integration of mental health into chronic disease prevention and health promotion. *Preventing Chronic Disease, 3*(2), A61. Available from URL: http://www.cdc.gov/pcd/issues/2006/apr/05_0215. htm.
14. Luoma, J. B., Martin, C. E., & Pearson, J. L. (2002). Contact with mental health and primary care providers before suicide: A review of the evidence. *American Journal of Psychiatry, 159*(6), 909–916.
15. PAHO/WHO. (2017). *Mental health without borders.* Retrieved 12 Feb 2019 from https://www.paho.org/us/index.php?option=com_content&view=featured&lang=en
16. Padmanathan, P., & De Silva, M. J. (2013). The acceptability and feasibility of task-sharing for mental healthcare in low and middle-income countries: A systematic review. *Social Science & Medicine, 97*, 82–86.
17. Patel, V., Boyce, N., Collins, P. Y., Saxena, S., & Horton, R. (2011). A renewed agenda for global mental health. *Lancet (London, England), 378*(9801), 1441–1442. https://doi.org/10.1016/S0140-6736(11)61385-8.
18. Olfson, M., Blanco, C., Wang, S., Laje, G., & Correll, C. U. (2014). National trends in the mental health care of children, adolescents, and adults by office-based physicians. *JAMA Psychiatry, 71*(1), 81–90.
19. World Health Organization. (2019). *Mental disorders prevention, promotion and management.* https://www.who.int/mental_health/publications/disorders_prevention_promotion/en/. Retrieved 13 Feb 2019.
20. World Health Organization. (2013). *Mental health action plan 2013–2020.* Available from URL: http://apps.who.int/iris/bitstream/10665/89966/1/9789241506021_eng.pdf
21. World Health Organization. (2017a). *mhGAP training manuals for the mhGAP intervention guide for mental, neurological and substance use disorders in non-specialized health settings-version 2.0* (for field testing).
22. World Health Organization. (2017b, July). Retrieved 27 Aug 2017 from http://www.who.int/mental_health/mhgap/July_2017_mhGAP_Newsletter.pdf?ua=1
23. World Health Organization, World Organization of National Colleges, Academies, & Academic Associations of General Practitioners/Family Physicians. (2008). *Integrating mental health into primary care: A global perspective.* World Health Organization.
24. World Health Organization. (2007). *Mental health policy, planning and service development information sheet: The optimal mix of services* [Internet]. http://www.who.int/mental_health/policy/services/2_OptimalMixofServices_Infosheet.pdf
25. World Health Organization. (2003). *WHO health policy and service guidance package: Organization of services for mental health.* Geneva: WHO.
26. World Health Organization. (2002). *Prevention and promotion in mental health.* https://apps.who.int/iris/bitstream/handle/10665/42539/9241562161.pdf;jsessionid=6574FC5F0189ED63744C2796F51C4704?sequence=1. Retrieved 13 Feb 2019.
27. Steel, Z., Silove, D., Phan, T., & Bauman, A. (2002). Long-term effect of psychological trauma on the mental health of Vietnamese refugees resettled in Australia: a population-based study. *Lancet, 360*(9339), 1056–1062.

28. Cabassa, L. J., Lagomasino, I. T., Dwight-Johnson, M., Hansen, M. C., & Xie, B. (2008). Measuring Latinos' perceptions of depression: A confirmatory factor analysis of the Illness Perception Questionnaire. *Cult Divers Ethn Minor Psychol, 14*(4), 377–384.
29. Hines-Martin, V., Malone, M., Kim, S., & Brown-Piper, A. (2009). Barriers to mental health care access in an African American population. *Issues Ment Health Nurs, 24*(3), 237–256.
30. Carson, N. J., Vesper, A., Chen, C.-n., & Lê Cook, B. (2014). Quality of follow-up after hospitalization for mental illness among patients from racial-ethnic minority groups. *Psychiatr Serv, 65*(7), 888–896.
31. Straiton, M. L., Powell, K., Reneflot, A., & Diaz, E. (2015). Managing mental health problems among immigrant women attending primary health care services. *Health Care Women Int, 37*(1), 118–139.
32. Mihaljević, S., Vuksan-Ćusa, B., Marčinko, D., Koić, E., Kušević, Z., & Jakovljević, M. (2011). Spiritual well-being, cortisol, and suicidality in Croatian war veterans suffering from PTSD. *J Relig Health, 50*(2), 464–473.
33. Vogel, D. L., Heimerdinger-Edwards, S. R., Hammer, J. H., & Hubbard, A. (2011). "Boys don't cry": examination of the links between endorsement of masculine norms, self-stigma, and help-seeking attitudes for men from diverse backgrounds. *J Couns Psychol, 58*(3), 368–382.
34. Murray, S. B., & Skull, S. A. (2005). Hurdles to health: immigrant and refugee health care in Australia. *Aust Health Rev, 29*(1), 25.
35. Patel, V., Saxena, S., Lund, C., Thornicroft, G., Baingana, F., Bolton, P., Chisholm, D., Collins, P. Y., Cooper, J. L., Eaton, J., Herrman, H., Herzallah, M. M., Huang, Y., Jordans, M. J. D., Kleinman, A., Medina-Mora, M. E., Morgan, E., Niaz, U., Omigbodun, O., Prince, M., Rahman, A., Saraceno, B., Sarkar, B. K., De Silva, M., Singh, I., Stein, D. J., Sunkel, C., & UnÜtzer, J. Ü. (2018). The Lancet Commission on global mental health and sustainable development. *Lancet, 392*(10157), 1553–1598.
36. Chisholm, D., James, S., Sekar, K., Kishore Kumar, K., Srinivasa Murthy, R., Saeed, K., & Mubbashar, M. (2000). Integration of mental health care into primary care. *Br J Psychiatry, 176*(6), 581–588.
37. Braun, R., Catalani, C., Wimbush, J., Israelski, D., & Bullen, C. (2013). Community health workers and mobile technology: a systematic review of the literature. *PLoS One, 8*(6), e65772.
38. Kok, M. C., Kane, S. S., Tulloch, O., Ormel, H., Theobald, S., Dieleman, M., Taegtmeyer, M., Broerse, J. E. W., & de Koning, K. A. M. (2015). How does context influence performance of community health workers in low- and middle-income countries? Evidence from the literature. *Health Res Policy Syst, 13*(1).
39. (2017). Treating depression where there are no mental health professionals. *Bull World Health Organ, 95*(3), 172–173.

Chapter 8
Governance, Diplomacy and Politics – Diversity and Lifespan

Sabine Bährer-Kohler, A. Soghoyan, and K. Gasparyan

Key Points

- Good governance refers to, for example, responsibility, accountability, participation, and sustainability [40].
- Governance, diplomacy and politics can build up trust and understanding, awareness and knowledge, and can encourage solving the current challenges or can try to eliminate or reduce difficulties in this context and to promote solutions and improvements.
- Challenges related to diversity and lifespan are:

  1. To build up better awareness-raising about diversity over the lifespan.
  2. To pursue and integrate greater knowledge and reflection about diversity over the lifespan, to promote and support prevention & mental health promotion, and to avoid stigmatization [3].
  3. To involve more national and international agencies, institutions, organizations and associations, for example with petitions, statements, programs and applications.
  4. Clear outcomes and action points for challenges Nos. 1–3 should be documented [45].

- Knowledge and understanding about diversity during the lifespan has to be implemented in education, public education, higher education and training [10].

(continued)

S. Bährer-Kohler (✉)
Dr. Bährer-Kohler & Partner, Basel, Switzerland

International University of Catalonia (UIC), Barcelona, Spain
e-mail: sabine.baehrer@datacomm.ch

A. Soghoyan · K. Gasparyan
Yerevan State Medical University, Yerevan, Armenia

© The Author(s) 2019
S. Bährer-Kohler, B. Bolea-Alamanac (eds.), *Diversity in Global Mental Health*,
SpringerBriefs in Psychology, https://doi.org/10.1007/978-3-030-29112-9_8

- Diversity must find better ways in education and training across all stages of mental health and psychiatry training [27].
- Governance, diplomacy and politics have great potential to solve challenges related to diversity over the lifespan.
- The United Nations, as a global organization that brings together its member states, has great potential to solve challenges in aspects of diversity, lifespan and mental health in a global context.
- Other organizations, federations and associations like the World Psychiatric Association (WPA) have great potential to solve challenges of diversity, lifespan, and global mental health.
- Individuals, NGOs and foundations have great potential to influence challenges.
- Networks, cooperation and collective actions are always required [44].
- Power hereby remains one of the key concepts of international politics [2].
- Guidelines with proven standards, markers and high-quality investigations for diversity, lifespan and global mental health are required.

8.1 Introduction

The topic of the booklet is diversity, lifespan and global mental health in a broad context. This chapter will focus on the transformation and on possibilities of international and/or national governance, diplomacy and politics to support and to develop solutions, to achieve improvements and to protect human rights in the context of diversity, lifespan and global mental health. At the beginning of this chapter basics will be defined, which means specifying the three terms – governance, diplomacy and politics in particular, and identifying current tasks or challenges and/or future tasks in the context of diversity and lifespan.

With several scientific analyses and utility analyses, it was possible to cluster and focus (a) on main areas, (b) on specific topics, and (c) to categorize forgotten topics.

Such a process is not devoid of certain criticisms such as subjectivity, but with more than 100 analyzed publications, this concept has a sound and solid background.

Awareness of many topics was the starting point of the elevator, the collection of solid and scientific data with the inclusion of qualitative studies and their analysis was the ground floor; further analysis and utility analysis was the first floor, before reaching the upper floors. The attic allowed a perspective for the whole topic to identify the significant challenges [44], and ways to reach specific aims, embedded in a changing world with transformational changes across global issues [43].

The results include multiple possibilities and, as always, networking, national and international cooperation and collective actions are required [44]. More than 55% of countries in any WHO region and more than 75% of Eastern Mediterranean, South East Asian, Western Pacific and European countries reported that they have updated their policy/plan in the last 5 years [51].

8.2 Content

8.2.1 Clarification of Terms

Governance is often used as an organizing concept that guides administrators as administrative practices shift ([34], p. 2). However, no single and exhaustive definition of 'good governance' exists, nor a delimitation of its scope that would command universal acceptance [40].

The World Bank concluded that 'good governance' entails sound public sector management (efficiency, effectiveness and economy), accountability, exchange and free flow of information (transparency), and a legal framework for development (justice, respect for human rights and liberties) [34]. Furthermore, the Commission on Human Rights in its resolution 2000/64 identified the key attributes and facets of good governance as:

- transparency
- responsibility
- accountability
- participation
- responsiveness (to the needs and desires of the people) [40].

Diplomacy: To build up trust is a very important task in governance issues and in diplomacy. The European Commission stated that public diplomacy refers to the long-lasting process whereby a country [or an entity] seeks to build trust and understanding by engaging with a broader foreign public beyond the governmental relations [8].

Traditional forms of diplomacy are increasingly supplemented with forms of public diplomacy in the consultation, exchange, negotiation and governance of political geographies and constellations of world order with national and international harmony, and national and global disorder [15, 17].

Global health diplomacy should bring together the disciplines of public health, international affairs, management, law and economics, and focuses on negotiations that manage the global policy environment for health, to identify and understand key current, future changes and challenges impacting global public health, and to build capacity to support the necessary collective responses, innovations and actions [47].

Politics are the activities of a state, government or other institution, often combined with the process of making decisions that apply to the members of a specific group.

Power remains hereby one of the key concepts of international politics, state power is related to national power [2].

The power of the United Nations is often controversially discussed [33], for example related to the regular budget, which has doubled over the past two decades to $5.4bn, and to the annual UN expenditure, which is 40 times higher than it was in the early 1950s. The United Nations is a unique international organization founded in 1945, with 193 Member States at present. All missions and work of the United Nations are guided by the purposes and principles contained in its founding charter, which was signed on 26 June 1945 [35]. Here, Article 1 of Chap. 1 about purposes and principles underlines that international peace and security and effective collective measures for the prevention and removal of threats to the peace are fundamental.

8.3   Diversity and Lifespan

Diversity and diverse identities coexisting within the same society, in the same country, on the same continent, are very often viewed as problematic for social, economic and political development [9]. However, cultural diversity in a diverse society can enrich innovation and creativity. Diversity can enrich countries, spirits and national character. Diversity and its expression could determine individual nations, national and international components and future aspects. Discussion and critical reflection about diversity are a remarkable opportunity to focus on the potential of diversity [4]. Involvement, engagement and participation in such discussions and critical reflections are required.

Furthermore, a challenge facing humanity is the extension of life expectancy worldwide, which in turn has an effect on the nature of various chronic and non-chronic illnesses, which require global readiness for the provision of new service forms and investments.

But up to now, around the globe, great challenges exist related to aspects of diversity over the lifespan:

A. *To build up more awareness – to receive benefits*

After detailed analysis, it must be concluded that the awareness related to diversity over the lifespan is not sufficient. For example, [26] (PricewaterhouseCoopers International) conducted a global, cross-industry survey with business, diversity& inclusion (D&I), and human resources (HR) leaders. One result was that 48% of respondents still agree or strongly agree that diversity is a barrier. A current publication of Mc Kinsey & Company [19] concluded that growing awareness of the business case for inclusion and diversity exists, but progress has been slow.

The key features of successful awareness, for example with awareness-raising campaigns, are very well known ([7], p. 6 ff.; [5]). Objectives and target groups must be defined, tools and channels must be identified, and partners or networks must be identified and selected at the beginning of and during such processes.

B. *To pursue and integrate greater knowledge and reflection – to receive benefits*

Studies
- Scientific databanks, for example the [46, 25], OECD iLibrary 2018 [20], and other databanks published up to October 2018 had only a limited number of studies or results related to diversity and lifespan.

- Diversity and lifespan is a complex topic, far more sound information and current scientific data are required.
- In addition, further global guidelines on searching for scientific information [31] are needed.
- In a next step to select data, the data-information-knowledge-wisdom (DIKW) hierarchy or pyramid, can be a useful model [28].

Documentation and publications

Currently, International Labour Organization (ILO), Pan American Health Organization (PAHO), World Health Organization (WHO) and United Nations (UN), for example, have remarkable documentation; here a brief selection:

- ILO [12]. ILO Action Plan for Gender Equality 2018–21.
- ILO [13]. Gender, Equality and Diversity Branch (GED).
- PAHO/WHO [21]. Cultural Diversity and Health.
- UN [36]. World Day for Cultural Diversity for Dialogue and Development | 21 May.
- UN [37]. Universal Declaration on Cultural Diversity.
- UNESCO [39]. UNESCO Universal Declaration on Cultural Diversity.
- WHO [48]. Gender, equity and human rights. Health and sexual diversity. FAQ on Health and Sexual Diversity- An Introduction to Key Concepts (2016).
- WHO [49]. Gender and health.
- WHO [50]. Health, environment and climate change. Human health and biodiversity.

Surveys

Surveys to examine opinions related to diversity and lifespan can be important and significant. Here a few examples:

- The Diversity Engagement Survey [41]. Twelve thousand and eighty (12,080) University of Rochester faculty, staff, trainees, and students completed this survey in 2016.
- The Board Diversity Survey, a survey which was conducted in 2017 among 300 board members/ internal directors and C-suite executives at U.S. companies with at least $50 million in annual revenue and at least 1000 employees [11].
- The global diversity & inclusion survey, a global, cross-industry survey [26].
- The Diversity Engagement Survey (DES) by Person et al. [24] to measure how well academic medical centers are responding to the diversity of their communities.

Books

There are current books, which are especially related to specific aspects of diversity, i.e. by [29], Parry and McCarthy [23], and [18] (Eds.).

There are books in this field, which are especially related to diversity, mental health, mental health promotion, and with inclusion to avoid stigmatization, i.e. by Parekh [22], Levin and Becker [16], Khanlou and Pilkington (Eds.) [14], and [42].

A current book related to mental health across lifespan is edited by Steen and Thomas [30]. The book with the title: Mental Health across the Lifespan: a Handbook covers specific aspects of diversity, such as ethnicity, gender and age groups.

Education
Knowledge and understanding of diversity during the lifespan has to be implemented in education, public education, higher education and training [10]. Diversity is a stable reality, and culturally responsive teaching respectively education is a pedagogy of inclusion and acceptance [6] and responsive teaching in higher education institutions, for example, where diversity is daily present both on the supplier and customer side [1]. Diversity must find better ways in education and training on issues of culture, bias, and health disparities across all stages of mental health training and psychiatry training [27].

To summarize Basics and scientific publications exist as fragments, but for the complex areas and many-faceted factors related to *diversity over the lifespan and global mental health*, an overall conception and guidelines or comprehensive, embracing publications especially from international institutions are still missing and required. This could be a future-oriented promotion and investigation for diversity over the lifespan and global mental health, with possible impacts at all levels.

C. *To support and involve national & international agencies and institutions*

The overall results of the analysis show there are multiple possibilities, but national and international networks, cooperation and collective actions are always essential [44]. To support the United Nations, officially three main areas are documented.

- The United Nations offers to work on a voluntary basis to help contact lawmakers, to raise funds, to organize meetings and to find partners for joint projects. And further, to organize or participate in UN-related events in schools and in other settings.
- As an inter-governmental body, the UN relies primarily on Member States but also welcomes grassroots initiatives to promote its work, its concepts and ideas.
- Or to donate money [38].

To push issues and to support topics, the structures, conceptions, conditions and the working structures of the United Nations have to be known. The United Nations has specific main organs with specific functions and regulations. With, for example, the General Assembly, Security Council Economic and Social Council, and the Trusteeship Council. Every one of the 193 member states has specific competencies and possibilities.

Every single person, every organization, every association, etc. has in principle the possibility to force topics within a change process. Change is often about advocacy [32], often with petitions, statements, programs and applications, for example.

- With awareness of issues that should be changed, influenced or supported better.
- With analysis, aims, tasks, and expected outcomes.
- Afterwards, petitions and statements, etc. have to be formulated. With networks, partners, national and/or international partners and the best methods to achieve the targeted aims.

Clear outcomes and action points should always be documented [45] to reach a positive impact at all or at most levels.

8.4 Remarks & Discussion

Basics and outstanding scientific publications exist as fragments. Nevertheless, for the complex areas and many-faceted factors related to diversity over the lifespan and global mental health, overall conceptions or guidelines, or comprehensive, embracing publications especially from an international institution such as the United Nations, the World Health Organization, the World Bank or from other international bodies, are missing and urgently required. As documented in other chapters of this booklet, diversity over the lifespan has great influence and impact.

The United Nations, as the global organization with 193 member states, has great potential to respond to challenges in aspects of diversity and lifespan.

Besides international bodies, there are other organizations like the WPA, World Federation for Mental Health (WFMH), International Psychogeriatric Association (IPA), which have possibilities as a multiplier, and as organizations of experts. For example, the World Psychiatric Association (WPA) a global association of national psychiatric societies and with their beginnings in 1950 [53], aimed to increase the knowledge and skills necessary for work in the field of mental health and the care for the mentally ill [52], WPA tries to increase knowledge, competencies and skills about mental disorders and how they can be prevented and treated. The WPA has members who are experts with competency about global mental health, and it has experts with competencies related to diversity and global mental health.

As noted in the Mental Health Atlas [51], the policy, plan and laws for mental health should comply with international human rights conventions, such as the Convention on the Rights of Persons with Disabilities (CRPD). The majority of difficulties are related to the lack of proper awareness and knowledge in different countries. Various countries have their own specificities. It is accepted that international agencies, such as the ones mentioned above, are largely capable of creating universal instruments that are used on a global level. However, their implementation is influenced by objective and subjective factors, including bureaucracy, societal resistance or retardation and related stigma.

8.5   Conclusion

- Good governance refers to responsibility, accountability, participation, and sustainability, for example [40].
- Governance, diplomacy, and politics can build up trust and understanding, awareness and knowledge, and can help to solve the current challenges or reduce or eliminate difficulties in the context of diversity over the lifespan, and global mental health.
- Challenges related to diversity and lifespan are:

  To build up better awareness about diversity over the lifespan and prevention & mental health promotion, to encourage more knowledge about it, to avoid stigmatization, and to support and involve national and international agencies and institutions with, for example, petitions, statements, programs and applications. Clear outcomes and action points should be documented hereby [45].

- Governance, diplomacy and politics have great potential to respond to challenges.
- The United Nations, as a global organization that brings together its member states, has great potential to solve challenges in aspects of diversity, lifespan and global mental health.
- Other organizations, federations and associations such as the WPA have great potential to meet challenges of diversity, lifespan, and global mental health.
- Networks, cooperation and collective actions are always required [44].
- Individuals, NGOs and foundations have great potential to influence challenges.
- Power remains hereby one of the key concepts [2].

Future Tasks
- To bring issues of diversity over the lifespan to the attention of stakeholders and responsible institutions.
- To utilize existing networks, professional networks, alliances and governmental structures.
- To strengthen the communication between the structures of international policy makers and local stakeholders. One of the best umbrella organization could be WPA, which has member societies in more than 120 countries worldwide and could initiate implementation of various levels.
- To strengthen leadership and governance in order to develop well-defined policies and critical resources. To monitor and identify gaps, failures and lessons learned from implemented policies/plans.
- To utilize formal and informal structures of international and national bodies, associations etc.

- An overall conception and guidelines or comprehensive, embracing publications, especially from international institutions or international bodies, are still lacking and required. This could be a future-orientated promotion and investigation for diversity over the lifespan and global mental health, in a global context.
- To provide guidelines with proven standards, benchmarks and high-quality investigations for diversity, lifespan and global mental health are required.
- Knowledge and understanding about diversity during the lifespan has to be implemented in education, public education, higher education and training [10].
- Diversity must find better ways in education and training across all stages of mental health and psychiatry training [27].
- Recommend packages of protocols and guidelines to groups of countries, which have similar social-cultural and financial profiles recommended by the World Bank and WHO. This could help them create or review their Mental Health policies in the context of their cultural, economic and even political sensitivities.
- Process control and evidence-based analysis are required.

References

1. Aigare, A., Thomas, P. L., & Koyumdzhieva, T. (2011). *Diversity management in higher education institutions: Key motivators* (Bachelor Thesis in Business Administration). http://www.diva-portal.org/smash/get/diva2:426378/FULLTEXT02.pdf. Retrieved 5 Oct 2018.
2. Al-Rodhan, N. (2018). The seven capacities of states: A meta-geopolitical framework. *The Georgetown Journal of International Affairs.* https://www.georgetownjournalofinternationalaffairs.org/online-edition/2018/3/7/the-seven-capacities-of-states-a-meta-geopolitical-framework. Retrieved 27 Sept 2018.
3. Bährer- Kohler, S. (2017). *Global mental health.* Prevention and promotion. https://www.springer.com/de/book/9783319591223. Retrieved 11 Oct 2018.
4. Bolkus, N. (2018). *Political aspects of diversity - Social justice in a changing Australia.* https://www.dss.gov.au/our-responsibilities/settlement-services/programs-policy/a-multicultural-australia/programs-and-publications/1995-global-cultural-diversity-conference-proceedings-sydney/political-aspects-of-diversity/political-aspects-of-diversity-social. Retrieved 1 Oct 2018.
5. EC- European Commission. (2013). *Strategies for improving participation in and awareness of adult learning: European Guide.* Luxembourg, Publications Office of the European Union. In ELINET (2015, p. 9). http://www.eli-net.eu/fileadmin/ELINET/Redaktion/user_upload/The_key_features_of_successful_awareness_raising__campaigns_10-15_LM_ELINET.pdf. Retrieved 1 Oct 2018.
6. Egbo, B. (2018). *Culturally responsive teaching: A pedagogy of inclusion.* http://www.oecd.org/education/school/7-4th-Forum-EGBO.pdf. Retrieved 5 Oct 2018.
7. ELINET- European Literacy Policy Network (ELINET). (2015). *The key features of successful awareness raising campaigns.* http://www.eli-net.eu/. www.eli-net.eu/fileadmin/ELINET/Redaktion/user_upload/The_key_features_of_successful_awareness_raising__campaigns_10-15_LM_ELINET.pdf. Retrieved 6 Oct 2018.

8. EU - European Commission. (2014). *Public diplomacy (working definition)*. https://europa.eu/capacity4dev/pd-cd/wiki/public-diplomacy-working-definition. Retrieved 27 Sept 2018.
9. Gerring, J., Hoffman, M., & Zarecki, D. (2016). The diverse effects of diversity on democracy. *The British Journal of Political Science (BJPolS), 48*(2), 283–314. https://www.cambridge.org/core/journals/british-journal-of-political-science/article/div-classtitlethe-diverse-effects-of-diversity-on-democracydiv/6D33A5A58ADD41BAAF9D6551600360C9. Retrieved 1 Oct 2018.
10. Guo, Y. (2012). Diversity in public education: Acknowledging immigrant parent knowledge. *Canadian Journal of Education/Revue canadienne de l'éducation, 35*(2), 120–140.
11. Harvard Law School Forum on Corporate Governance and Financial Regulation. (2017). *2017 Board Diversity Survey*. https://corpgov.law.harvard.edu/2017/12/19/2017-board-diversity-survey/. Retrieved 1 Oct 2018.
12. ILO- International Labour Organization. (2018a). *ILO Action Plan for Gender Equality 2018–21*. https://www.ilo.org/gender/Informationresources/WCMS_645402/lang%2D%2Den/index.htm. Retrieved 4 Oct 2018.
13. ILO- International Labour Organization. (2018b). *Gender, Equality and Diversity Branch (GED)*. https://www.ilo.org/gender/lang%2D%2Den/index.htm. Retrieved 4 Oct 2018.
14. Khanlou, N., & Pilkington, B. (Eds.). (2015). *Women's mental health*. https://www.springer.com/la/book/9783319173252. Retrieved 5 Oct 2018.
15. Kissinger, H. (2014). *World order*. London: Penguin Press.
16. Levin, B. L., & Becker, M. A. (Eds.). (2010). *A public health perspective of Women's mental health*. https://www.springer.com/us/book/9781441915252. (Retrieved 5.10.18).
17. Loughborough University. (2018). *Centre for the Study of International Governance*. Research. Diplomacy and International Governance. http://www.lboro.ac.uk/departments/phir/research/research-centres/csig/diplomacy-and-international-governance/. Retrieved 27 Sept 2018.
18. Mansour, N., & Wegerif, R. (Eds.). (2013). *Science education for diversity. Theory and practice*. https://www.springer.com/us/book/9789400745629. Retrieved 5 Oct 2018.
19. Mc Kinsey & Company. (2018). *Delivering through diversity*. https://www.mckinsey.com/~/media/mckinsey/business%20functions/organization/our%20insights/delivering%20through%20diversity/delivering-through-diversity_full-report.ashx. Retrieved 1 Oct 2018.
20. OECD. (2018). *OECD iLibrary is the online library of the Organisation for Economic Cooperation and Development (OECD)*. www.oecd-ilibrary.org. Retrieved 1 Oct 2018.
21. PAHO/WHO. (2018). *Cultural diversity and health*. https://www.paho.org/hq/index.php?Itemid=4016&lang=en.8. Retrieved 4 Oct 2018.
22. Parekh, R. (Ed.). (2014). *The Massachusetts General Hospital textbook on diversity and cultural sensitivity in mental health*. https://www.springer.com/us/book/9781461489177. Retrieved 5 Oct 2018.
23. Parry, E., & McCarthy, J. (Eds.). (2017). *The Palgrave handbook of age diversity and work*. https://link.springer.com/book/10.1057/978-1-137-46781-2#about. Retrieved 5 Oct 2018.
24. Person, S. D., Jordan, C. G., Allison, J. J., et al. (2015). Measuring diversity and inclusion in academic medicine: The diversity engagement survey (DES). *Academic Medicine, 90*(12), 1675–1683. https://www.ncbi.nlm.nih.gov/pmc/articles/PMC5823241/. Retrieved 4 Oct 2018.
25. Pubmed. (2018). *Search diversity lifespan*. https://www.ncbi.nlm.nih.gov/pubmed/?term=diversity+lifespan. Retrieved 1 Oct 2018.
26. PWC. (2018). *Global diversity & inclusion survey*. https://www.pwc.com/gx/en/services/people-organisation/global-diversity-and-inclusion-survey.html. Retrieved 1 Oct 2018.
27. Rao, S., How, P. C., & Ton, H. (2018). Education, training, and recruitment of a diverse workforce in psychiatry. *Psychiatric Annals, 48*(3), 143–148. https://ucdavis.pure.elsevier.com/en/publications/education-training-and-recruitment-of-a-diverse-workforce-in-psyc. Retrieved 5 Oct 2018.
28. Rowley, J. (2007). The wisdom hierarchy: Representations of the DIKW hierarchy. *Journal of Information and Communication Science, 33*(2), 163–180. http://journals.sagepub.com/doi/10.1177/0165551506070706. Retrieved 1 Oct 2018.

29. Schönwälder, K., Petermann, S., Hüttermann, J., et al. (2016). *Diversity and contact. Immigration and social interaction in German cities.* https://www.palgrave.com/de/book/97811375 86025#aboutBook. Retrieved 5 Oct 2018.

30. Steen, M., & Thomas, M. (2015). *Mental health across the lifespan: A handbook.* Rotledge. https://books.google.fr/books?id=sQepCgAAQBAJ&pg=PR15&lpg=PR15&dq=diversity+lifespan+global+mental+health+books&source=bl&ots=N1_UPhotBI&sig=SJmJRInUeS_luuM2R6FxPeWL0WQ&hl=de&sa=X&ved=2ahUKEwjIrIHrjO_dAhVKIMAKHQC5COYQ6AEwAXoECAgQAQ#v=onepage&q=diversity%20lifespan%20global%20mental%20health%2. Retrieved 5 Oct 2018.

31. Students- University Utrecht. (2018). *Guidelines on Searching for Scientific Information.* students.uu.nl/sites/default/files/ucu_guidelines_for_searching_for_scientific_information.doc. Retrieved 1 Oct 2018. Or https://students.uu.nl/en

32. TDH. (2018). *For children, their rights and equitable development.* https://www.terredeshommes.org/. Retrieved 4 Oct 2018.

33. The Guardian. (2015). *70 years and half a trillion dollars later: what has the UN achieved?* https://www.theguardian.com/world/2015/sep/07/what-has-the-un-achieved-united-nations. Retrieved 1 Oct 2018.

34. UN- United Nations. (2006). *Definition of basic concepts and terminologies in governance and public administration.* http://unpan1.un.org/intradoc/groups/public/documents/un/unpan022332.pdf. Retrieved 27 Sept 2018.

35. UN- United Nations. (2018a). *Overview.* http://www.un.org/en/sections/about-un/overview/. Retrieved 27 Sept 2018.

36. UN- United Nations. (2018b). *World day for cultural diversity for dialogue and development | 21 May.* http://www.un.org/en/events/culturaldiversityday/. Retrieved 4 Oct 2018.

37. UN- United Nations. (2018c). *Universal declaration on cultural diversity.* http://www.un-documents.net/udcd.htm. Retrieved 4 Oct 2018.

38. UN- United Nations. (2018d). *Fact sheet: What the UNITED NATIONS does and what you can do to help.* https://visit.un.org/sites/visit.un.org/files/FS_What_the_UN_does_How_u_can_help_March2013.pdf. Retrieved 4 Oct 2018).

39. UNESCO. (2018). *UNESCO Universal Declaration on Cultural Diversity.* http://portal.unesco.org/en/ev.php-URL_ID=13179&URL_DO=DO_TOPIC&URL_SECTION=201.html. Retrieved 4 Oct 2018.

40. UN- OHCHR. (2018). *Good governance and human rights.* https://www.ohchr.org/en/issues/development/goodgovernance/pages/goodgovernanceindex.aspx. Retrieved 27 Sept 2018.

41. University of Rochester. (2018). *Diversity engagement survey.* https://www.rochester.edu/diversity/survey/. Retrieved 1 Oct 2018.

42. White, R. G., Jain, S., Orr, D. M. R., & Read, U. (Eds.). (2017). *The palgrave handbook of sociocultural perspectives on global mental health.* https://www.palgrave.com/gb/book/9781137395092. Retrieved 5 Oct 2018.

43. World Economic Forum. (2018a). *Mapping global transformations.* https://www.weforum.org/about/transformation-maps. Retrieved 27 Sept 2018.

44. World Economic Forum. (2018b). *Improving the state of the world.* https://www.weforum.org/our-impact. Retrieved 27 Sept 2018.

45. World Economic Forum. (2018c). *How do we do our work?* https://www.weforum.org/about/how-does-the-forum-do-its-work. Retrieved 4 Oct 2018.

46. World Bank. (2018). *Databank.* http://databank.worldbank.org/data/databases/page/1/orderby/popularity/direction/desc?qterm=diversity%20. Retrieved 1 Oct 2018.

47. WHO- World Health Organization. (2018a). *Trade, foreign policy, diplomacy and health.* Global Health Diplomacy. http://www.who.int/trade/diplomacy/en/. Retrieved 27 Sept 2018.

48. WHO- World Health Organization. (2018b). *Gender, equity and human rights. Health and sexual diversity.* FAQ on Health and Sexual Diversity- An Introduction to Key Concepts. (2016). http://www.who.int/gender-equity-rights/news/health-sexual-diversity/en/. Retrieved 4 Oct 2018.

49. WHO- World Health Organization. (2018c). *Gender and health.* http://www.who.int/news-room/fact-sheets/detail/gender. Retrieved 4 Oct 2018.
50. WHO- World Health Organization. (2018d). *Health, environment and climate change.* Human health and biodiversity. http://apps.who.int/gb/ebwha/pdf_files/WHA71/A71_11-en.pdf. Retrieved 4 Oct 2018.
51. Mental Health Atlas 2017. (2018). *WHO publication*, Geneva. http://www.who.int/mental_health/evidence/atlas/mental_health_atlas_2017/en/ Retrieved 12 Nov 2018.
52. WPA- World Psychiatric Association (2018a). *About the world psychiatric association.* http://www.wpanet.org/detail.php?section_id=5&content_id=4. Retrieved 6 Oct 2018.
53. WPA- World Psychiatric Association. (2018b). *History of the world psychiatric association.* http://www.wpanet.org/detail.php?section_id=5&content_id=44. Retrieved 6 Oct 2018.

Conclusion

Sabine Bährer-Kohler and Blanca Bolea-Alamanac

Promoting mental health is an integral part of the United Nations Sustainable Development Agenda. "Ensuring healthy lives and promoting the well-being at all ages is essential to sustainable development" [12]. Well-being includes dimensions like living standard, health, mental health, freedom, personal and community relationships, peace, and security [3].

This integration of mental health is from our point of view necessary, because mental disorders account for one of the largest and fastest growing categories of the burden of numerous diseases worldwide [8]. Scientific data have shown repeatedly that mental disorders can affect approximately one in four people [13], regardless country of origin.

Around the world approximately 450 million people suffer from such mental diseases as documented by WHO as far back as 2001. Today globally, an estimated 300 million people are affected by depression about 60 million people worldwide are affected by a bipolar affective disorder, about 23 million people worldwide are affected by schizophrenia, and approximately 50 million people have dementia [16].

In low- and middle-income countries, between 76% and 85% of all individuals with mental disorders receive no treatment for their disorder. In high-income countries, between 35% and 50% of all individuals with mental disorders are in a similar situation [16].

S. Bährer-Kohler (✉)
Dr. Bährer-Kohler & Partner, Basel, Switzerland

International University of Catalonia (UIC), Barcelona, Spain
e-mail: sabine.baehrer@datacomm.ch

B. Bolea-Alamanac
University of Toronto/Centre for Addiction and Mental Health, Toronto, ON, Canada

© The Author(s) 2019
S. Bährer-Kohler, B. Bolea-Alamanac (eds.), *Diversity in Global Mental Health*,
SpringerBriefs in Psychology, https://doi.org/10.1007/978-3-030-29112-9

This booklet about global mental health and diversity, lifespan, gender, treatment, service and access, prevention and promotion, governance and politics documents and summarizes relevant scientific data from observations, studies and research projects. Based on these data every chapter ends with a summary of well explained proposals and future tasks.

Additionally, this booklet acknowledges that many challenges in the context of *Global Mental Health* still exist and that these challenges can be met in effective and sustainable ways.

This booklet aims to influence decision-makers world-wide to meet these challenges and fill the gaps in mental health care.

Put the spotlight on mental health: One of the most important missions of this booklet is to bring mental illness and mental health care "out of the shadows", as [7] and others published a few years ago. We need to start talking more about mental health and this conversation needs to include individuals affected by mental illness, service providers, scientists and experts in the field, managers, politicians and other stakeholders in order to bring clarity and structure to future interventions, not only at the service level but also at a societal level. In this context, the interface between diversity and mental health, is very relevant. An effort was made to document extensively the main facts of this complex relationship in this booklet.

Better decisions: As co-editors we face the challenge of encouraging better decision making in mental health. The United Nations [11] states that informed and proper decisions can be made through

- "Collecting relevant information-
- Conducting situation analysis and making pertaining considerations based on best possible ratio risk/effectiveness and minimal level in the use of force-
- Identifying priorities-
- Identifying a coherent course of action;
- Translate the selected course of action into a plan in line with the strategic and operational guidance, plans and orders and respectful of the roles and mandated tasks of the other mission components and actors."

To convey this the booklet collected information, analyzed it and identified priorities. However, there is still a lot of work to do and multiple decisions to be made. Stakeholders, mental health workers, specialists, mental health professionals and allied staff in the mental health field, are all responsible for implementing change. Media including new social media, has a responsibility and a relevant role in breaking down misconceptions and myths [10], incorrect information about mental illness is not conducive to change in social, cultural and legal perceptions of mental health.

Decisions-stigma: Firm action to reduce stigmatization is required. Stigma of *mental illness* exists, worldwide, and is still a huge barrier for affected people and their families. Stigma operates in various ways in society: it is internalized by individuals, and is attributed by health and social professionals [1]. If affected people cannot reach services, if tolerance in society for mental health concerns and disease does not exist in a form, that allows the individual to access and demand mental health care, the circle for excellence in care including prevention, diagnosis, therapy, service structures and service access will turn around. Efforts to mitigate stigma through policy, public campaigns and by providing specific mental health training to healthcare professionals at all levels world-wide may be effective strategies to reach this goal [1]. Fighting stigma should include giving objective and evidence-based information on mental illnesses as well as providing positive representations of psychological health in the media, avoiding stereotypes that promote unhealthy behaviours such as domestic violence.

Decisions-economic support and investigations: Firm action is required to improve financial support for mental health services and research in the mental health sector. "Nobody should be missing out on mental health care because of the cost," said Dr Shekhar Saxena, the former Director of the Department of Mental Health and Substance Abuse (MSD) at the World Health Organization's Headquarters Office [15]. Current government expenditure on mental health is less than 1 US$ per capita in low and lower middle income countries whereas some high-income countries spend more than US$ 80 [15]. In the European Union only approximately 2.8% of the health budget was dedicated to mental health according to the EU Commission [6]. We should reflect on these data, particularly considering how promotion of mental wellbeing and prevention of mental illness specifically can improve global health.

Improving global focus:
In general, *Mental Health* promotion requires a global focus. We should perceive mental health as an international issue that requires cooperation across borders. Existing professional networks can be experienced global and national players and agents of change, stakeholders and agencies, are all important for *Global Mental Health*.

Action, empowerment and change:
The promotion and training of resilience in the health context is important, because a lack of resilience as a resource for successful coping might indicate a need for support during treatment [4]. Resilience is also an important factor in the prevention of mental illness and promotion of mental wellbeing. Historically, people with lived experience of mental illness lacked a voice ([18], p. 2). An important key message to guide action is that "people should be empowered to promote their own health, interact effectively with health services and be active partners in managing disease" ([17] in [18], p. 1).

Mental health care and education in mental wellbeing should be a priority with national and global attention as documented by Bird et al. [2], and by Giliberti and NAMI [5], the National Alliance on Mental Illness, which is the US nation's largest grassroots mental health organization.

WHO's Mental Health Action Plan 2013–2020 offers an example of the genesis of this increasing commitment by governments to enhance the priority given to mental health within their health and public policy [9] and recognizes universally the essential role of mental health in achieving better health for all people [16].

As co-editors we aspire to put diversity in the map as a key aspect integrated in the future of global mental health projects and global mental health working groups. To that effect, we sincerely hope this booklet will help to promote the human rights of people with mental health conditions and psychosocial disabilities all over the world [14].

Global health should be an international endeavor, in order to achieve better health worldwide, we must care about global mental health.

References

1. Ahmedani, B. K. (2011). Mental health stigma: Society, individuals, and the profession. *Journal of Social Work Values and Ethics, 8*(2), 41–416. https://www.ncbi.nlm.nih.gov/pmc/articles/PMC3248273/. Retrieved 14 Mar 2019.
2. Bird, P., Omar, M., Victor, D., et al. (2011). Increasing the priority of mental health in Africa: Findings from qualitative research in Ghana, South Africa, Uganda and Zambia. *Health Policy and Planning, 26*(5, 1), 357–365. https://academic.oup.com/heapol/article/26/5/357/741363. Retrieved 14 Mar 2019.
3. Eger, R. J., & Maridal, J. H. (2015). A statistical meta-analysis of the wellbeing literature. *International Journal of Wellbeing, 5*(2), 45–74. https://doi.org/10.5502/ijw.v5i2.4. https://internationaljournalofwellbeing.org/index.php/ijow/article/viewFile/364/477. Retrieved 14 Mar 2019.
4. Färber, F., & Rosendahl, J. (2018). The association between resilience and mental health in the somatically Ill. A systematic review and meta-analysis. *Deutsches Ärzteblatt International, 115*(38), 621–627. https://doi.org/10.3238/arztebl.2018.0621. https://www.aerzteblatt.de/int/archive/article/200713/The-association-between-resilience-and-mental-health-in-the-somatically-ill-a-systematic-review-and-meta-analysis. Retrieved 19 Mar 2019.
5. Giliberti, M. (2018). *Improving mental health should be a national priority.* https://www.nami.org/Blogs/From-the-CEO/February-2018/Improving-Mental-Health-Should-Be-a-National-Prior. Retrieved 14 Mar 2019.
6. Mental Health Europe. (2017). *10 things that you should know about mental health.* https://mhe-sme.org/wp-content/uploads/2017/12/10-things-you-should-know-1.pdf. Retrieved 13 Mar 2019.
7. Mnookin, S. (2016). *Out of the shadows: Making mental health a global development priority.* Washington, DC: World Bank Group. http://documents.worldbank.org/curated/en/2016/04/26281016/out-shadows-making-mental-health-global-development-priority. Retrieved 13 Mar 2019.
8. OECD. (2019). *Mental health.* http://www.oecd.org/health/mental-health.htm. Retrieved 4 Mar 2019.
9. Saxena, S., Funk, M., & Chisholm, D. (2014). WHO's Mental Health Action Plan 2013-2020: What can psychiatrists do to facilitate its implementation? *World Psychiatry, 13*(2), 107–109. https://www.ncbi.nlm.nih.gov/pmc/articles/PMC4102273/. Retrieved 4 Mar 2019.
10. Srivastava, K., Chaudhury, S., Bhat, P. S., et al. (2018). Media and mental health. *Indian Journal of Psychiatry, 27*(1), 1–5. https://www.ncbi.nlm.nih.gov/pmc/articles/PMC6198586/. Retrieved 19 Mar 2019.

11. UN- United Nations. (2015). *Decision making process.* http://dag.un.org/bitstream/handle/11176/387397/Decision%20making%20process.pdf?sequence=3&isAllowed=y. Retrieved 04 Mar 2019.
12. UN- United Nations. (2019). *Goal 3: Ensure healthy lives and promote well-being for all at all ages.* https://www.un.org/sustainabledevelopment/health/. Retrieved 04 Mar 2019.
13. WHO- World Health Organization. (2001). *World health report.* Mental disorders affect one in four people. https://www.who.int/whr/2001/media_centre/press_release/en/. Retrieved 4 Mar 2019.
14. WHO- World Health Organization. (2017). *Mental health.* WHO launches training tools to promote human rights in mental health services. https://www.who.int/mental_health/en/. Retrieved 4 Mar 2019.
15. WHO- World Health Organization. (2018a). *Mental health: Massive scale-up of resources needed if global targets are to be met.* https://www.who.int/mental_health/evidence/atlas/atlas_2017_web_note/en/. Retrieved 14 Mar 2019.
16. WHO- World Health Organization. (2018b). *Mental disorders.* https://www.who.int/news-room/fact-sheets/detail/mental-disorders. Retrieved 04 Mar 2019.
17. WHO- World Health Organization- Regional Office for Europe. (2006). *Gaining health. The European strategy for the prevention and control of noncommunnicable diseases.* Copenhagen: WHO Regional Office for Europe. http://www.euro.who.int/InformationSources/Publications/Catalogue/20061003_1. Retrieved 19 Mar 2019.
18. WHO- World Health Organization- Regional Office for Europe. (2010). *User empowerment in mental health – a statement by the WHO Regional Office for Europe (2010).* http://www.euro.who.int/__data/assets/pdf_file/0020/113834/E93430.pdf. Retrieved 19 Mar 2019.

Index

A
Abortion, 23
Access, 90, 91
Access to care, xi, xii, 54–61
Adolescent pregnancy, 23, 26
Adolescents, 21, 23–26
Adult age, 21
Age, 20–23
American academy of pediatrics (AAP), 35, 36
Anti-bullying policies, 36, 37
Anxiety, 8–13, 15
Anxiety disorders, 24
Associations, 82–84
Autonomy, 31
Awareness, 78, 80, 83, 84

B
Barriers, 55, 58, 60
Belief system, 59
Binational integration initiative, 66–73
Bio-psycho-social factors, 31
Biology of mental illness, 2
Biomedicine, xii
Bipolar affective disorder, 89
Borders, 91
Burden, 9, 14–16, 66, 68, 73

C
Child and adolescent, 58
Childhood, 21
Clinical trials, 43, 45–47
Collaborative approaches, 38
Collective actions, 78, 82, 84

Community health, 66, 69, 71
Community health workers (CHW), 66–73
Conditions, vii
Cooperation, 78, 82, 84
Coping, 91
Cost, 91
Cultural adaptations, 46
Cultural diversity, 14, 16, 55

D
Decision makers, 26
Decisions, 90, 91
Dementia, 89
Department of Mental Health and Substance Abuse (MSD), 91
Depression, 8–13, 15, 24, 89
Diplomacy, 78–85
Disability, 9–11, 15
Disability-adjusted life years (DALYS), 9, 14
Diversity, 2, 3, 5, 20–26, 32–38, 42–48, 54–56, 66–73, 90, 92
Domestic violence, 24
Drug abuse, 9
DSM-5, 56

E
Education, 20, 21, 23, 82, 85
Empowerment, 91
Equity, vii
Ethics, 13, 14, 16
Ethnic aspects, 24
Ethnic minorities, 44, 46, 47
Ethnic paradigms, 46

© The Author(s) 2019
S. Bährer-Kohler, B. Bolea-Alamanac (eds.), *Diversity in Global Mental Health*,
SpringerBriefs in Psychology, https://doi.org/10.1007/978-3-030-29112-9

Printed in the United States
By Bookmasters